EAT

TO BEAT YOUR DIET FOR

SENIORS:

A RECENT SCIENCE GUIDE TO

MANAGE DISEASES AND LIVE

LONGER

H. Y. ABRAHAM

DISCLAIMER

The information provided in this book, "Eat to Beat Your Diet for Seniors: A Recent Science Guide to Manage Diseases and Live Longer," authored by H. Y. Abraham, is intended for informational purposes only. The author and publisher are not engaged in rendering medical, legal, financial, or other professional services. Any content within this book should not be considered a substitute for professional advice, diagnosis, or treatment. Readers are advised to consult with qualified healthcare professionals, nutritionists, or other experts regarding their specific health and dietary needs.

The author and publisher of this book disclaim any liability or responsibility for any adverse effects, consequences, or damages resulting from the use of the information presented herein. The dietary and nutritional recommendations provided in this book are based on current scientific knowledge and research available at the time of writing. However, nutritional science is continually evolving, and individual dietary needs can vary.

Readers should use their discretion and consult with professionals to make informed decisions about their diet and health. Every effort has been made to ensure the accuracy and completeness of the information presented in this book. Nevertheless, the author and publisher make no representations or warranties with respect to the accuracy or completeness of the contents and disclaim all warranties, express or

ACKNOWLEDGMENTS

I would like to express my heartfelt gratitude to the individuals and institutions who have contributed to the creation of this book, First and foremost, I extend my appreciation to the dedicated healthcare professionals and researchers whose work has paved the way for the valuable information contained in these pages. Your commitment to advancing our understanding of senior nutrition and health is truly commendable. I am deeply thankful to my family and friends for their unwavering support, encouragement, and patience throughout the writing process. Your belief in the importance of this book has been a source of inspiration. I would also like to express my gratitude to Mark L., whose meticulous editing and proofreading greatly enhanced the clarity and readability of this book. My sincere thanks go to Sarah V., Vegan for the exceptional cover design. I appreciate the assistance provided by Michael P in gathering and organizing the extensive research material that forms the foundation of this book.

Finally, my appreciation extends to the readers of this book. Your curiosity and dedication to improving your health and well-being through informed nutrition choices have motivated me to share this knowledge.

Thank you all for being a part of this journey to promote healthier and longer lives for seniors through the science of nutrition.

With heartfelt thanks,

H. Y. Abraham

PREFACE

As I embarked on the journey of writing "Eat to Beat Your Diet for Seniors: A Recent Science Guide to Manage Diseases and Live Longer," I was driven by a profound belief in the transformative power of nutrition. The quest to unravel the secrets of senior nutrition and its profound impact on health and longevity became a personal mission.

This book is a culmination of extensive research, a commitment to providing accurate and up-to-date information, and a sincere desire to empower seniors to take control of their health through dietary choices. It's a testament to the remarkable advancements in nutritional science and the boundless potential for seniors to live healthier, more fulfilling lives. Our journey begins with an exploration of the science behind senior nutrition. We delve into the fascinating world of recent discoveries that shed light on the intricate relationship between diet and health. Throughout these pages, you will find a wealth of knowledge, practical advice, and, most importantly, a sense of hope.

Seniors are a vibrant and diverse group, each with their unique stories, challenges, and aspirations. "Eat to Beat Your Diet for Seniors" is designed to be a comprehensive resource that meets you where you are on your health journey. Whether you seek solutions to manage specific health conditions, aspire to prevent illness, or simply wish to embrace a healthier lifestyle, this book is your guide. One of the key features of this book is the inclusion of monthly meal plans. These plans offer a structured approach to applying the principles of senior nutrition in your day-to-day life. They are crafted with care to provide a variety of delicious and nutritious options that cater to different tastes and dietary preferences. As we embark on this voyage through the science of senior nutrition, disease management, and longevity, remember that knowledge is your greatest ally.

This book aims to equip you with the understanding and tools to make informed choices about your diet and health. It is my hope that the insights shared here will inspire you to embrace a future filled with vitality, health, and joy. I invite you to explore the chapters that follow, engage with the meal plans, and, above all, take charge of your well-being. The path to a healthier and longer life begins with the choices you make today. Together, let's eat to beat our diets and thrive in the golden years.

With warm regards,

H. Y. Abraham.

INTRODUCTION

Welcome to "Eat to Beat Your Diet for Seniors: A Recent Science Guide to Manage Diseases and Live Longer." In the pages that follow, we embark on a journey of discovery—a journey that explores the profound impact of nutrition on the health and longevity of seniors. This book is your gateway to a world of knowledge, insights, and practical strategies designed to empower you on your path to healthier, more fulfilling golden years.

Seniorhood is a chapter of life defined by wisdom, experience, and the well-earned joys of retirement. It is a time to savor the fruits of a life well-lived. Yet, it can also bring its unique set of challenges, including health concerns that become more prominent with age. It is here, amid these challenges, that the importance of nutrition shines brighter than ever before.

The aging process affects our bodies in various ways, altering metabolism, nutrient absorption, and overall health. It is a time when dietary choices can play a pivotal role in either managing and preventing diseases or contributing to health decline. This book is your compass through these critical choices.

A Science-Based Approach

At the heart of this book lies a commitment to science-based nutrition. We will journey together through the latest research, exploring how dietary choices can influence health and longevity. The field of nutritional science is constantly evolving, and recent discoveries have reshaped our understanding of what constitutes a healthy diet, particularly for seniors.

A Guide Tailored to Seniors

This book is crafted with you, the senior reader, in mind. It recognizes your unique needs, preferences, and challenges. It provides guidance on how to navigate the intricate world of senior nutrition, offering practical steps that can be seamlessly integrated into your daily life.

You will find comprehensive advice on creating a senior-friendly kitchen, meal planning, and preparing nutritious, delicious meals. We understand that eating should be both a pleasure and a source of vitality. Therefore, we've included an extensive collection of recipes tailored to seniors' dietary requirements and designed to tantalize your taste buds.

Disease Management and Prevention

Disease management and prevention are central themes in this book. We explore how nutrition can complement medical treatments, offering strategies for managing specific health conditions. You will also uncover the power of proactive nutrition, learning how to prevent diseases through diet, and discovering foods and nutrients that can fortify your body against common health challenges.

Monthly Meal Plans

One distinctive feature of this book is the inclusion of monthly meal plans. These plans offer a structured and practical approach to applying the principles of senior nutrition. Each month provides a new set of meal ideas, accompanied by shopping lists and nutritional information. They are designed to take the guesswork out of meal planning and make healthy eating an enjoyable and achievable goal.

Your Journey Begins

Your journey through "Eat to Beat Your Diet for Seniors" begins now. Whether you are seeking solutions to manage specific health conditions, aspiring to prevent illness, or simply wishing to embrace a healthier lifestyle, this book is your trusted companion. It is a roadmap to better health, one founded on the latest scientific insights and tailored to your unique needs.

As we venture through the chapters that follow, remember that knowledge is your greatest ally. By the end of this book, you will possess the understanding and tools to make informed choices about your diet and health. Together, let's embark on a path to vitality, health, and joy in your golden years. Let's eat to beat our diets and thrive.

With warm regards,

H. Y. Abraham

CHAPTER 2: UNDERSTANDING SENIOR NUTRITION

In our journey to unlock the secrets of senior nutrition and its profound impact on health and longevity, understanding the unique nutritional needs of seniors is our starting point. The aging process brings about changes in the body's metabolism, nutrient absorption, and overall health. These changes necessitate a closer look at what constitutes a healthy diet for seniors.

2.1. The Science of Senior Nutrition

In our exploration of senior nutrition, it's crucial to lay a solid foundation by understanding the scientific principles that underpin this field. Senior nutrition is not a one-size-fits-all concept; it's a dynamic area of study shaped by the evolving science of aging and dietary research.

The Importance of Nutrition for Seniors

Nutrition has always been vital for health, but its significance takes on new dimensions as we age. For seniors, maintaining proper nutrition becomes instrumental in sustaining health, energy, and vitality. Here, we delve into why nutrition is a cornerstone of well-being for this demographic:

- **Supporting Bodily Functions:** Nutrients obtained through diet serve as the building blocks for essential bodily functions. These functions include cell repair, immune system strength, and maintaining vital organ health.

- **Disease Prevention and Management:** A well-balanced diet can help prevent or manage various health conditions commonly associated with aging, such as hypertension, diabetes, heart disease, and osteoporosis. The right nutrients can bolster the body's defenses against these conditions.

- **Enhancing Quality of Life:** Nutrition isn't just about physical health. It plays a significant role in mental and emotional well-being. The right diet can contribute to cognitive function, mood stability, and overall life satisfaction.

2.2 Recent Scientific Insights

The field of nutritional science is continually evolving, and recent breakthroughs have illuminated the unique dietary needs and challenges faced by seniors. It's crucial to stay informed about these insights, as they form the foundation of our dietary recommendations in this book:

1. **Tailored Nutritional Approaches:** Recent research has highlighted the importance of customized dietary plans for seniors. One-size-fits-all dietary advice may not be suitable, as individual needs can vary widely. Scientific studies now emphasize personalized nutritional approaches to address the specific health concerns of older adults.

2. **Understanding Nutrient Absorption:** Seniors may experience changes in their ability to absorb certain nutrients. For example, calcium absorption may decline, which is relevant for bone health. Understanding these changes helps us adapt dietary recommendations accordingly.

3. **The Role of Nutrient Timing:** Emerging research suggests that when you eat can be as important as what you eat. Exploring the timing of meals and fasting windows can be instrumental in managing health and metabolism in seniors.

4. **Gut Microbiota and Health:** The study of gut microbiota, the trillions of microorganisms residing in our digestive system, has revealed its profound impact on health. Recent insights show that maintaining a healthy gut microbiome through diet can benefit seniors by improving digestion, immune function, and overall well-being.

5. **Superfoods and Functional Foods:** Scientific research has identified certain foods, often referred to as "superfoods" or "functional foods," that offer exceptional health benefits. We will explore how incorporating these foods into the senior diet can contribute to enhanced well-being.

6. **Balancing Macronutrients:** Recent studies have emphasized the importance of a balanced intake of macronutrients—carbohydrates,

proteins, and fats. Understanding the role of each macronutrient in senior nutrition is essential for maintaining health and managing weight.

Throughout this book, we will incorporate these recent scientific insights into practical dietary guidance. It's our commitment to provide you with up-to-date, evidence-based information that empowers you to make informed choices about your diet and health.

As we proceed in our journey through senior nutrition, we will dive deeper into the specifics of nutrient requirements, disease management, and disease prevention. Together, we'll navigate the path to healthier and longer living, fueled by the latest scientific discoveries in the realm of nutrition.

2.3. Common Health Challenges for Seniors

As we age, our bodies undergo various changes that can make us more susceptible to certain health challenges. Understanding these common health issues is crucial for tailoring a diet that addresses the specific needs and concerns of seniors.

Overview of Health Challenges

Seniors may encounter a range of health challenges that can impact their quality of life and overall well-being. It's important to be aware of these conditions and how nutrition can play a role in their prevention and management:

1. **Cardiovascular Diseases:** Heart diseases, including hypertension (high blood pressure) and atherosclerosis (narrowing of arteries), become more prevalent with age. Nutrition choices can directly influence heart health, and we will explore dietary strategies to promote cardiovascular well-being.

2. **Diabetes:** Type 2 diabetes is a common concern among seniors. Proper nutrition can help manage blood sugar levels, and we will discuss the role of diet in preventing and controlling diabetes.

3. **Osteoporosis:** Bone health is a significant consideration for seniors, particularly postmenopausal women. Calcium and vitamin D intake, along with other nutrients, are pivotal in preventing osteoporosis.

4. **Cognitive Decline:** Age-related cognitive decline and conditions like Alzheimer's disease pose significant challenges. Emerging research suggests that certain nutrients and dietary patterns can support brain health and cognitive function.

5. **Arthritis:** Arthritis, characterized by joint pain and inflammation, often affects seniors. Nutritional choices can impact inflammation levels and help manage arthritic symptoms.

6. **Nutrient Deficiencies:** As we age, our bodies may have difficulty absorbing essential nutrients, leading to deficiencies. Understanding these challenges can guide dietary choices and the use of supplements when necessary.

2.4 Nutrition's Role in Managing Senior Health

Each of these health challenges presents unique dietary considerations. Nutrition can play a pivotal role in managing and preventing these conditions, offering seniors a path to improved health and well-being.

Throughout this book, we will explore specific dietary strategies and nutrient recommendations tailored to address these health challenges. By understanding the connection between nutrition and health, you will be better equipped to make informed choices that can contribute to a healthier and longer life.

Our journey through senior nutrition continues as we delve deeper into the essentials of senior nutrition, the significance of maintaining healthy body fat, and proactive nutrition approaches. Together, we'll navigate the path to optimal health and longevity, armed with knowledge and practical strategies.

CHAPTER 3: THE ESSENTIALS OF SENIOR NUTRITION

In our exploration of senior nutrition, it's crucial to lay a strong foundation by understanding the key components that make up a healthy and balanced diet for seniors. This chapter delves into the essentials of senior nutrition, providing you with the knowledge needed to make informed dietary choices that can lead to a healthier and longer life.

3.1. Balancing Macronutrients

In the world of senior nutrition, achieving a balanced intake of macronutrients—carbohydrates, proteins, and fats—is the cornerstone of a healthy diet. Properly balancing these nutrients not only supports overall well-being but also addresses specific health concerns that seniors may face.

Carbohydrates: The Energy Source

Carbohydrates are the body's primary source of energy. However, not all carbs are created equal. Seniors should focus on complex carbohydrates, which provide sustained energy and valuable fiber:

- **Whole Grains:** Whole grains like oats, brown rice, quinoa, and whole wheat pasta are excellent sources of complex carbohydrates. They provide lasting energy and contain essential nutrients like fiber, vitamins, and minerals.

- **Fruits and Vegetables:** These natural sources of carbohydrates not only offer energy but also supply essential vitamins and antioxidants. Opt for a colorful array of fruits and vegetables to benefit from a wide range of nutrients.

- **Legumes:** Beans, lentils, and chickpeas are rich in complex carbs and plant-based protein. They also provide fiber, which supports digestive health and helps manage blood sugar levels.

Proteins: Building Blocks for Health

Proteins are the building blocks of the body. They are essential for maintaining and repairing tissues, supporting immune function, and aiding in the production of enzymes and hormones. Seniors should focus on lean sources of protein:

- **Poultry:** Skinless poultry like chicken and turkey is a lean protein source. It provides essential amino acids without excess saturated fat.

- **Fish:** Fatty fish such as salmon, mackerel, and trout not only deliver protein but also heart-healthy omega-3 fatty acids. These fats support brain health and reduce inflammation.

- **Beans and Tofu:** For plant-based protein, turn to beans, lentils, tofu, and other soy products. They offer a protein boost along with fiber and various vitamins and minerals.

Fats: The Good, the Bad, and the Healthy

Fats are essential for overall health, including brain function and the absorption of fat-soluble vitamins. However, it's crucial to distinguish between healthy and unhealthy fats:

- **Healthy Fats:** Unsaturated fats found in avocados, nuts, seeds, and olive oil are beneficial for seniors. They support heart health and cognitive function.

- **Unhealthy Fats:** Saturated and trans fats, often found in fried foods and processed snacks, should be limited. These fats can contribute to heart disease and inflammation.

Balancing Act

Balancing macronutrients is a nuanced process, and the ideal balance can vary among individuals based on their health goals and medical conditions. Seniors are encouraged to work with healthcare professionals or registered dietitians to create personalized dietary plans that address their specific needs.

Understanding the role of each macronutrient in senior nutrition empowers you to make informed choices about your diet. As we continue our journey through senior nutrition, we'll explore the significance of micronutrients, hydration, and dietary fiber in supporting your health and longevity.

Micronutrients, which include vitamins and minerals, are the unsung heroes of senior nutrition. These essential compounds play a critical role in various bodily functions and are paramount for maintaining overall health and vitality in your senior years. Let's explore the key micronutrients that should be in the spotlight of your senior nutrition plan.

Calcium: Building Strong Bones

Calcium is a micronutrient that deserves special attention, especially for seniors. It is the primary mineral responsible for building and maintaining strong bones. Adequate calcium intake is vital in preventing osteoporosis and fractures, which become more common with age. Some excellent sources of calcium include:

- **Dairy Products:** Milk, yogurt, and cheese are well-known calcium-rich foods.

- **Fortified Plant-Based Milk:** For those who are lactose intolerant or follow a plant-based diet, fortified plant-based milk alternatives like almond, soy, or oat milk are good options.

- **Leafy Greens:** Dark, leafy greens such as kale, collard greens, and spinach are natural sources of calcium.

- **Tofu:** Calcium-set tofu is a versatile plant-based source of this mineral.

Vitamin D: The Sunshine Vitamin

Vitamin D plays a vital role in calcium absorption and bone health. It's often referred to as the "sunshine vitamin" because your skin can produce it when exposed to sunlight. However, many seniors may have reduced sun exposure or difficulty absorbing vitamin D from sunlight. Therefore, it's essential to include dietary sources and, if necessary, supplements:

- **Sun Exposure:** Spend some time outdoors in the sun, preferably during midday when UVB rays are most abundant. Consult with a healthcare professional to determine your specific sun exposure needs.

- **Dietary Sources:** Fatty fish like salmon and mackerel, fortified foods (such as fortified milk and cereals), and egg yolks contain vitamin D.

- **Supplements:** Your healthcare provider may recommend vitamin D supplements to ensure you meet your requirements.

Vitamin B12: Nerve Health and More

Vitamin B12 is essential for nerve health, red blood cell production, and DNA synthesis. Deficiency can lead to anemia and neurological issues, which can be more common in seniors. Sources of vitamin B12 include:

- **Animal Products:** Meat, fish, eggs, and dairy products are rich in vitamin B12.

- **Fortified Foods:** Some fortified plant-based foods like breakfast cereals, plant-based milk, and nutritional yeast contain vitamin B12. This is particularly important for seniors following vegetarian or vegan diets.

Folate: Cell Division and More

Folate, also known as vitamin B9, is crucial for cell division and the formation of DNA. It can help prevent certain birth defects and supports overall health. Foods rich in folate include:

- **Leafy Greens:** Spinach, kale, and collard greens are excellent natural sources.

- **Legumes:** Beans, lentils, and chickpeas provide folate along with protein and fiber.

- **Fortified Foods:** Some grains and cereals are fortified with folate.

Vitamin C: Immune Support and More

Vitamin C is an antioxidant that supports the immune system, promotes wound healing, and aids in the absorption of iron from plant-based sources. Seniors can find vitamin C in:

- **Citrus Fruits:** Oranges, grapefruits, lemons, and limes are well-known sources.

- **Berries:** Strawberries, blueberries, and raspberries are rich in vitamin C.

- **Bell Peppers:** Red and green bell peppers contain more vitamin C than most fruits.

A Comprehensive Approach

Micronutrients are like puzzle pieces that fit together to maintain health. To ensure you're getting a well-rounded intake of these essential nutrients, aim for a diverse and colorful diet that includes a variety of fruits, vegetables, lean proteins, and whole grains. For personalized guidance on micronutrient intake, consult with a registered dietitian or healthcare provider.

As we delve deeper into senior nutrition, we'll continue to explore the vital role of hydration, dietary fiber, and other key factors in maintaining your health and well-being.

In the realm of senior nutrition, maintaining proper hydration is often an underestimated yet vital component of overall health. The importance of staying adequately hydrated cannot be overstated, especially for seniors. In this section, we explore the significance of hydration for senior health and provide guidance on how to ensure you remain well-hydrated.

Why Hydration Matters for Seniors

Proper hydration is essential for people of all ages, but it holds particular relevance for seniors due to several factors:

- **Reduced Thirst Sensation:** As we age, our bodies may become less efficient at signaling thirst. This can lead to a decreased desire to drink fluids even when dehydration is imminent.

- **Altered Kidney Function:** Aging can affect kidney function, potentially reducing the body's ability to concentrate urine and conserve water.

- **Medications:** Many seniors take medications that can have diuretic effects or alter fluid balance, increasing the risk of dehydration.

- **Increased Risk of Heat-Related Illnesses:** Seniors are often more susceptible to heat-related conditions, such as heat stroke, which can be exacerbated by dehydration.

Signs of Dehydration

Recognizing the signs of dehydration is crucial for senior health. Common symptoms include:

- Dry mouth and dry skin

- Dark urine or infrequent urination

- Dizziness or lightheadedness

- Rapid heart rate

- Fatigue

- Confusion or irritability

If you experience any of these symptoms, it's essential to address your hydration immediately.

Hydration Strategies

To maintain proper hydration, consider the following strategies:

- **Regular Water Intake:** Aim to drink water throughout the day, even if you don't feel thirsty. Sip water with meals and between meals.

- **Hydrating Foods:** Many fruits and vegetables have high water content and can contribute to your daily hydration. Examples include watermelon, cucumbers, and oranges.

- **Monitor Urine Color:** Pay attention to the color of your urine. Pale or light yellow urine is a good indicator of adequate hydration, while dark yellow or amber urine may signal dehydration.

- **Limit Dehydrating Beverages:** Reduce the consumption of beverages with diuretic effects, such as caffeinated and alcoholic drinks.

- **Stay Cool:** During hot weather or physical activity, take extra precautions to stay hydrated. Drink water and avoid excessive sun exposure.

- **Consult Your Healthcare Provider:** If you have specific medical conditions or take medications that affect hydration, consult with your healthcare provider for personalized hydration recommendations.

Remember that individual hydration needs can vary based on factors like climate, activity level, and overall health. It's essential to listen to your body and make conscious efforts to stay hydrated. Proper hydration is a simple yet powerful way to support your overall well-being and vitality as a senior.

As we continue our exploration of senior nutrition, we'll delve into the importance of dietary fiber, digestive health, and other factors that contribute to your health and longevity.

3.4. Fiber and Digestive Health

Fiber is a dietary powerhouse, and its role in senior nutrition cannot be overstated. It offers a multitude of health benefits, particularly in maintaining digestive health and overall well-being. In this section, we'll explore the significance of dietary fiber and how it contributes to digestive health for seniors.

Understanding Dietary Fiber

Dietary fiber is a type of carbohydrate found in plant-based foods that our bodies cannot digest. Instead, it passes through the digestive system relatively intact, providing a range of health benefits. There are two primary types of dietary fiber:

1. **Soluble Fiber:** This type of fiber dissolves in water and forms a gel-like substance in the digestive tract. It can help lower cholesterol levels and stabilize blood sugar.

2. **Insoluble Fiber:** Insoluble fiber does not dissolve in water and adds bulk to stool, aiding in regular bowel movements. It helps prevent constipation and promotes digestive regularity.

Digestive Health Benefits of Fiber

For seniors, maintaining digestive health becomes increasingly important. Dietary fiber plays several critical roles in promoting a healthy digestive system:

1. **Preventing Constipation:** Insoluble fiber adds bulk to stool, making it easier to pass. This helps prevent constipation, a common issue among older adults.

2. **Supporting Bowel Regularity:** Fiber encourages regular bowel movements, reducing the risk of discomfort and bloating associated with irregularity.

3. **Diverticular Disease Prevention:** A high-fiber diet may lower the risk of diverticulosis and diverticulitis, conditions characterized by pouches in the colon that can become inflamed.

4. **Hemorrhoid Prevention:** Fiber helps prevent the development of hemorrhoids, painful swollen veins around the rectum.

5. **Maintaining Gut Health:** Dietary fiber supports the growth of beneficial gut bacteria, contributing to a healthy gut microbiome. A well-balanced gut microbiome is linked to improved overall health.

Sources of Dietary Fiber

You can find dietary fiber in a variety of foods, and it's essential to incorporate a range of fiber-rich options into your diet. Some excellent sources of dietary fiber include:

- Whole grains like oats, whole wheat, and brown rice.

- Fruits such as apples, pears, and berries.

- Vegetables like broccoli, carrots, and spinach.

- Legumes, including beans, lentils, and chickpeas.

- Nuts and seeds like almonds, chia seeds, and flaxseeds.

Gradual Increase and Hydration

If you're not accustomed to a high-fiber diet, it's essential to increase your fiber intake gradually to allow your digestive system to adjust. Additionally, drink plenty of water when increasing fiber intake to help prevent digestive discomfort.

Dietary fiber is a nutritional ally in promoting digestive health and overall well-being for seniors. By incorporating fiber-rich foods into your diet, you can support regular bowel movements, prevent digestive issues, and contribute to a healthy gut microbiome.

3.5 Building Balanced Senior Meals

As we delve deeper into the essentials of senior nutrition, it's crucial to understand how to translate nutritional principles into balanced and satisfying meals. In this section, we'll explore the art of creating well-rounded senior meals that provide the nutrients and energy needed for a healthy and vibrant life.

The Components of a Balanced Meal

A balanced meal should encompass a variety of nutrients to support overall health and well-being. When planning senior meals, aim to include the following components:

1. **Lean Protein:** Protein is essential for muscle maintenance and overall health. Incorporate lean protein sources such as poultry, fish, beans, tofu, and low-fat dairy into your meals.

2. **Whole Grains:** Whole grains like brown rice, quinoa, and whole wheat pasta provide sustained energy and essential nutrients like fiber, vitamins, and minerals. They are excellent choices for seniors.

3. **Colorful Vegetables:** Vegetables offer a wealth of vitamins, minerals, and antioxidants. Opt for a variety of colorful options, such as leafy greens, carrots, bell peppers, and broccoli, to ensure a broad spectrum of nutrients.

4. **Fruits:** Fruits are natural sources of vitamins, fiber, and natural sugars. Enjoy a range of fruits like berries, oranges, apples, and bananas for added nutritional variety.

5. **Healthy Fats:** Incorporate healthy fats from sources like avocados, nuts, seeds, and olive oil to support brain health and overall well-being.

6. **Dairy or Dairy Alternatives:** If you consume dairy, choose low-fat or fat-free options. For those following a dairy-free diet, select fortified plant-based milk alternatives like almond, soy, or oat milk.

Portion Control and Nutrient Density

While focusing on nutrient variety, it's also essential to consider portion control. Seniors often have different energy needs compared to younger individuals, so be mindful of serving sizes. Additionally, prioritize nutrient-dense foods, which provide a high concentration of essential nutrients for the calories they contain.

Meal Planning Tips for Seniors

Here are some practical meal planning tips to create balanced and nutritious meals:

1. **Plan Ahead:** Plan your meals in advance to ensure you have a variety of nutrient-rich foods on hand.

2. **Use Herbs and Spices:** Enhance the flavor of your meals with herbs and spices instead of excessive salt, which can impact blood pressure.

3. **Stay Hydrated:** Don't forget to include water as part of your meal. Proper hydration is crucial for overall health.

4. **Mindful Eating:** Pay attention to portion sizes and avoid eating in front of the television or while distracted. Mindful eating can help you enjoy your meals and prevent overeating.

5. **Balanced Snacking:** If you snack between meals, opt for healthy choices like yogurt, whole-grain crackers with hummus, or fresh fruit.

Building balanced senior meals is an art that combines nutritional wisdom with culinary creativity. By including a variety of nutrient-rich foods in your meals and paying attention to portion sizes, you can ensure that your diet supports your health and vitality in your senior years.

3.6 The Role of Healthy Body Fat

While discussions of body fat often revolve around weight management, it's essential to recognize that not all body fat is created equal. In this section, we'll explore the concept of healthy body fat and its role in senior nutrition and overall well-being.

Understanding Healthy Body Fat

Body fat serves several critical functions in the body, including:

1. **Energy Storage:** Fat stores energy that the body can utilize during times of reduced food intake or increased energy demands.

2. **Insulation:** Fat acts as insulation, helping to regulate body temperature and protect vital organs.

3. **Hormone Production:** Fat tissue produces hormones that play a role in various bodily functions, including metabolism and immune system regulation.

The Importance of Healthy Body Fat for Seniors

Maintaining an appropriate amount of body fat is essential for seniors for several reasons:

1. **Insulation and Temperature Regulation:** Adequate body fat helps insulate against temperature extremes, which can be crucial for seniors who may be more sensitive to temperature changes.

2. **Energy Reserve:** Healthy body fat serves as an energy reserve, which can be especially valuable during illness or periods of decreased appetite.

3. **Hormone Production:** Fat tissue produces hormones, some of which are essential for metabolic and immune system health. Ensuring a healthy balance of body fat contributes to hormonal balance.

The Difference between Healthy and Unhealthy Body Fat

It's crucial to differentiate between healthy body fat and excess body fat associated with health risks. The distribution of body fat can also impact health:

1. **Subcutaneous Fat:** This type of fat is located just under the skin and serves as insulation. It's generally considered healthy in moderate amounts.

2. **Visceral Fat:** Visceral fat surrounds internal organs and is associated with health risks when it accumulates in excessive amounts. High levels of visceral fat are linked to conditions like heart disease and diabetes.

Balancing Body Composition

For seniors, achieving and maintaining a healthy body composition is key. This involves not only managing body fat but also preserving and building lean muscle mass. Strength training exercises, along with a balanced diet, can support muscle health and contribute to a favorable body composition.

Healthy body fat plays a multifaceted role in senior health. It provides insulation, energy reserves, and hormonal support. Maintaining a balance between healthy body fat and lean muscle mass is crucial for overall well-being

CHAPTER 4: NUTRITION FOR DISEASE MANAGEMENT AND PREVENTION

In this pivotal chapter, we embark on a journey to explore the profound impact of nutrition on disease management and prevention for seniors. By understanding how specific dietary choices can influence various health conditions, you'll gain the knowledge needed to take proactive steps toward a longer, healthier life.

4.1 Heart Health: Nourishing Your Cardiovascular System

Your heart is at the center of your well-being, and maintaining its health is paramount, especially for seniors. In this section, we'll explore the intricate relationship between nutrition and heart health, unveiling dietary strategies and heart-healthy foods that can support your cardiovascular system.

Understanding Heart Disease Risk

Heart disease remains a significant concern for seniors, but proactive dietary choices can make a profound difference. It's vital to recognize the risk factors associated with heart disease, including:

- High blood pressure (hypertension)

- High cholesterol levels

- Obesity or excess body weight

- Diabetes

- Smoking

- Sedentary lifestyle

- Family history of heart disease

The Role of Nutrition in Heart Health

Diet plays a central role in managing and preventing heart disease. By adopting heart-healthy eating habits, you can mitigate risk factors and enhance your cardiovascular well-being. Here are some key dietary considerations:

1. Fruits and Vegetables: Embrace a colorful array of fruits and vegetables rich in antioxidants and fiber. These foods can help lower blood pressure, reduce cholesterol levels, and protect against heart disease.

2. Whole Grains: Opt for whole grains like oats, quinoa, and whole wheat, which provide essential fiber and nutrients that support heart health.

3. Lean Proteins: Choose lean protein sources such as skinless poultry, fish, legumes, and tofu. These options are lower in saturated fat, which can contribute to heart disease.

4. Healthy Fats: Incorporate healthy fats from sources like avocados, nuts, seeds, and olive oil. These fats can help lower bad cholesterol (LDL) and reduce inflammation.

5. Limit Sodium: Reduce your sodium intake by minimizing processed and high-sodium foods. Lowering salt intake can help manage blood pressure.

6. Watch Sugar Intake: Be mindful of added sugars in your diet, as excessive sugar consumption can contribute to obesity and diabetes, both of which impact heart health.

7. Portion Control: Pay attention to portion sizes to avoid overeating and excessive calorie consumption.

8. Hydration: Stay well-hydrated with water, as dehydration can strain your heart.

Mindful Eating for Heart Health

Mindful eating is a valuable practice for heart health. By savoring your meals, you're more likely to recognize fullness cues and avoid overindulging. Additionally, mindful eating can reduce stress, which is linked to heart disease.

Heart health is a lifelong journey, and nutrition is a fundamental aspect of this path. By nourishing your cardiovascular system with heart-healthy foods and adopting dietary practices that mitigate risk factors, you can take substantial steps toward a heart-healthy future.

For seniors living with diabetes or at risk of developing it, effective blood sugar management is a top priority. In this section, we'll delve into the intricate relationship between nutrition and diabetes management, providing guidance on how to achieve and maintain stable blood sugar levels through mindful eating and balanced meals.

Understanding Diabetes in Seniors

Diabetes is a metabolic disorder characterized by elevated blood sugar levels. There are two primary types of diabetes:

1. **Type 1 Diabetes:** This form of diabetes is typically diagnosed in childhood or young adulthood and results from the body's inability to produce insulin.

2. **Type 2 Diabetes:** Type 2 diabetes is more common in adults and is often linked to lifestyle factors, including diet and physical activity. In this type, the body becomes resistant to insulin or doesn't produce enough to maintain normal blood sugar levels.

The Role of Nutrition in Diabetes Management

Diet plays a pivotal role in managing both type 1 and type 2 diabetes. For seniors, adopting a diabetes-friendly diet can help stabilize blood sugar levels and reduce the risk of complications. Here are essential dietary considerations:

1. Carbohydrate Management: Carbohydrates significantly impact blood sugar levels. Focus on complex carbohydrates with a low glycemic index, such as whole grains, legumes, and non-starchy vegetables. Monitor portion sizes to control carbohydrate intake.

2. Balanced Meals: Aim for balanced meals that include lean protein sources, healthy fats, and fiber-rich carbohydrates. This combination can help prevent blood sugar spikes.

3. Fiber Intake: Dietary fiber is beneficial for diabetes management as it slows the absorption of sugar and promotes stable blood sugar levels. Include high-fiber foods like vegetables, fruits, whole grains, and legumes in your diet.

4. Sugar and Sweeteners: Minimize added sugars and sugary beverages. Artificial sweeteners can be an option, but use them in moderation.

5. Portion Control: Pay attention to portion sizes to avoid overeating and to regulate calorie intake.

6. Regular Meals: Consistency in meal timing can help stabilize blood sugar levels. Aim to eat meals and snacks at roughly the same times each day.

7. Monitor Blood Sugar: Regularly monitor your blood sugar levels as advised by your healthcare provider to track your progress and make necessary adjustments to your diet.

8. Hydration: Stay well-hydrated with water, as dehydration can affect blood sugar levels.

Meal Planning and Diabetes

Meal planning is a valuable tool for diabetes management. It allows you to control carbohydrate intake, monitor portion sizes, and maintain balanced meals. Working with a registered dietitian can be particularly helpful in developing personalized meal plans to meet your specific dietary needs and diabetes goals.

Diabetes management through nutrition is a dynamic journey that involves careful attention to food choices, portion sizes, and overall meal planning. By adopting a diabetes-friendly diet, you can take proactive steps to stabilize blood sugar levels and minimize the impact of diabetes on your daily life. In the upcoming sections, we'll explore nutrition's role in managing other common health conditions affecting seniors.

4.3 Bone Health: Strengthening Your Skeletal System

Maintaining strong and healthy bones is a vital aspect of senior nutrition. In this section, we'll explore the significance of bone health for seniors, emphasizing the role of nutrition in preserving and fortifying your skeletal system.

Understanding Bone Health for Seniors

Aging can bring about changes in bone density and structure, making seniors more susceptible to conditions like osteoporosis and fractures. Here are some key aspects to consider:

1. Calcium: Calcium is a cornerstone of bone health. Adequate calcium intake is essential for maintaining bone density and strength. Dairy products, fortified foods, and leafy green vegetables are excellent sources of calcium.

2. Vitamin D: Vitamin D is crucial for calcium absorption. Sunlight is a natural source of vitamin D, and it's also found in fatty fish, fortified foods, and supplements.

3. Magnesium: Magnesium supports bone health by aiding in calcium absorption. You can find magnesium in nuts, seeds, whole grains, and leafy greens.

4. Protein: Protein is essential for muscle and bone health. Incorporate lean protein sources like poultry, fish, beans, and tofu into your diet.

5. Vitamin K: Vitamin K plays a role in bone metabolism and calcium regulation. Leafy green vegetables like kale and spinach are rich in vitamin K.

6. Avoid Excessive Salt and Caffeine: High salt and caffeine intake can lead to calcium loss from bones. Limit your consumption of salty and caffeinated foods and beverages.

7. Stay Active: Weight-bearing exercises, such as walking and strength training, can help maintain bone density and muscle mass.

8. Avoid Smoking and Excess Alcohol: Smoking and excessive alcohol consumption can negatively impact bone health. If you smoke, seek support to quit, and consume alcohol in moderation.

Dietary Practices for Strong Bones

Incorporating bone-healthy foods and dietary practices into your daily life is crucial for preserving skeletal strength. Consider the following:

1. Dairy or Dairy Alternatives: If you consume dairy, choose low-fat or fat-free options. For those following a dairy-free diet, select fortified plant-based milk alternatives like almond, soy, or oat milk.

2. Leafy Greens: Consume plenty of leafy green vegetables like kale, collard greens, and spinach to increase your intake of bone-strengthening nutrients.

3. Nuts and Seeds: Almonds, chia seeds, and flaxseeds are rich in calcium and magnesium, making them excellent choices for bone health.

4. Fortified Foods: Some foods, such as fortified cereals and plant-based milk, are enriched with calcium and vitamin D, making them convenient options for bolstering bone health.

Maintaining strong and healthy bones is essential for seniors to enjoy an active and independent lifestyle. By focusing on bone-friendly foods and dietary practices, you can fortify your skeletal system and reduce the risk of fractures and bone-related conditions.

4.4 Brain Health: Nourishing Cognitive Function

Preserving cognitive function is a top priority for seniors, and nutrition plays a pivotal role in supporting brain health. In this section, we'll explore the complex relationship between nutrition and cognitive vitality, unveiling dietary strategies and brain-boosting foods to maintain and enhance your cognitive function.

The Significance of Brain Health

Cognitive health encompasses memory, attention, problem-solving, and overall mental well-being. Maintaining cognitive function is crucial for seniors to lead fulfilling and independent lives. Consider these factors:

1. Cognitive Decline: Age-related cognitive decline is common but not inevitable. Certain lifestyle factors, including diet, can influence the rate and extent of cognitive decline.

2. Brain Diseases: Neurodegenerative diseases like Alzheimer's and Parkinson's can affect cognitive function in seniors. While there is no cure, nutrition may play a role in reducing the risk of these conditions.

3. Mental Wellness: Good mental health is closely connected to cognitive function. Proper nutrition can help support emotional well-being and reduce the risk of conditions like depression and anxiety.

Nutrients for Brain Health

Several nutrients have been linked to cognitive health and brain function. Incorporating these nutrients into your diet can be beneficial for your brain:

1. Omega-3 Fatty Acids: Omega-3s, found in fatty fish like salmon and walnuts, have anti-inflammatory properties and may help maintain cognitive function.

2. Antioxidants: Antioxidant-rich foods like berries, leafy greens, and colorful vegetables protect brain cells from oxidative stress and inflammation.

3. B Vitamins: B vitamins, particularly B6, B9 (folate), and B12, are essential for brain health and may reduce the risk of cognitive decline. They can be found in whole grains, legumes, leafy greens, and lean proteins.

4. Vitamin D: Vitamin D may play a role in cognitive health. Exposure to sunlight and vitamin D-rich foods like fatty fish and fortified dairy products can support brain function.

5. Curcumin: Curcumin, a compound found in turmeric, has anti-inflammatory and antioxidant properties and may benefit cognitive health.

6. Hydration: Proper hydration is crucial for cognitive function. Dehydration can impair focus and cognitive performance.

Dietary Strategies for Cognitive Health

Adopting a brain-healthy diet involves more than individual nutrients. It's about overall dietary patterns. Consider these strategies:

1. Mediterranean Diet: The Mediterranean diet, rich in fruits, vegetables, whole grains, olive oil, and fish, has been associated with cognitive health and a reduced risk of cognitive decline.

2. DASH Diet: The Dietary Approaches to Stop Hypertension (DASH) diet, which emphasizes fruits, vegetables, lean proteins, and low-fat dairy, may benefit both brain and heart health.

3. Mindful Eating: Mindful eating practices can help prevent overeating and promote healthy food choices, supporting both cognitive and emotional well-being.

4. Stay Socially Active: Social interaction is essential for cognitive health. Maintaining connections with friends and loved ones can support brain function.

Nourishing your cognitive function through nutrition is a proactive step toward maintaining mental clarity and well-being as you age. By incorporating brain-boosting foods and dietary practices into your daily life, you can promote cognitive vitality and enhance your quality of life.

4.5 Weight Management: Achieving and Maintaining a Healthy Weight

Weight management is a multifaceted aspect of senior nutrition that goes beyond aesthetics. Maintaining a healthy weight is essential for overall health and well-being. In this section, we'll explore the science-backed strategies for achieving and sustaining a healthy weight through balanced eating, portion control, and mindful dietary choices.

Understanding the Importance of Healthy Weight

Excess body weight can have a profound impact on senior health, contributing to various health issues, including:

1. Heart Disease: Obesity is a risk factor for heart disease, increasing the likelihood of hypertension, high cholesterol, and heart attacks.

2. Type 2 Diabetes: Obesity is closely linked to type 2 diabetes, as excess body fat can lead to insulin resistance.

3. Joint Problems: Carrying excess weight places additional stress on the joints, increasing the risk of osteoarthritis and joint pain.

4. Sleep Apnea: Obesity is a common cause of sleep apnea, a condition that disrupts sleep and can lead to other health issues.

5. Reduced Mobility: Obesity can limit mobility, making it harder to engage in physical activities and maintain independence.

The Science of Weight Management

Achieving and maintaining a healthy weight requires a balance between energy intake (calories consumed) and energy expenditure (calories burned). Here's how nutrition plays a vital role:

1. Caloric Balance: To lose weight, you must create a caloric deficit by consuming fewer calories than you burn. Conversely, to gain weight, you need a caloric surplus.

2. Balanced Meals: Focus on balanced meals that provide essential nutrients without excess calories. Incorporate lean proteins, whole grains, fruits, vegetables, and healthy fats.

3. Portion Control: Be mindful of portion sizes to avoid overeating. Use smaller plates and pay attention to hunger and fullness cues.

4. Mindful Eating: Mindful eating practices can help you develop a healthy relationship with food, recognizing true hunger and avoiding emotional eating.

5. Physical Activity: Combine a balanced diet with regular physical activity to support weight management. Strength training exercises can help preserve muscle mass.

6. Hydration: Stay well-hydrated with water to support metabolism and avoid confusing thirst with hunger.

Strategies for Sustainable Weight Management

Weight management is not about quick fixes but sustainable changes. Consider the following strategies:

1. Set Realistic Goals: Establish achievable weight loss or weight maintenance goals that align with your health and lifestyle.

2. Seek Support: Enlist the help of a healthcare provider or registered dietitian to create a personalized weight management plan.

3. Track Progress: Monitor your food intake, physical activity, and progress toward your goals. Keeping a food diary can be helpful.

4. Gradual Changes: Make gradual dietary changes rather than drastic restrictions. This promotes long-term adherence.

5. Emotional Eating: Identify emotional triggers for overeating and develop healthier coping strategies.

Achieving and maintaining a healthy weight is a crucial aspect of senior nutrition that contributes to overall well-being and quality of life. By adopting science-based strategies, making mindful dietary choices, and staying physically active, you can take control of your weight and promote a healthier, more vibrant senior life.

4.6 Proactive Nutrition: Guarding Against Common Ailments

Prevention is often the best medicine, and proactive nutrition can help you stay resilient against common health issues that affect seniors. In this section, we'll explore the role of nutrition in bolstering your immune system, preventing common ailments, and promoting overall well-being.

The Power of Immune Support

As you age, your immune system may weaken, making you more susceptible to infections and illnesses. Proper nutrition can fortify your immune system, reducing the risk of common ailments like colds, flu, and respiratory infections. Here's how:

1. Nutrient-Rich Foods: Consuming a variety of nutrient-rich foods, such as fruits, vegetables, whole grains, lean proteins, and healthy fats, provides the vitamins, minerals, and antioxidants essential for immune function.

2. Hydration: Staying well-hydrated with water supports all bodily functions, including immune responses.

3. Probiotics: Foods like yogurt, kefir, and fermented vegetables contain beneficial probiotics that promote a healthy gut microbiome, which is closely linked to immune health.

4. Adequate Protein: Protein is essential for the production of antibodies and immune cells. Include lean protein sources in your diet.

5. Antioxidants: Antioxidants found in foods like berries, citrus fruits, and leafy greens combat free radicals and reduce inflammation, supporting immune function.

6. Vitamins and Minerals: Vitamins like vitamin C, vitamin D, and zinc play critical roles in immune health. Ensure your diet includes foods rich in these nutrients.

Preventing Respiratory Illnesses

Respiratory infections can be particularly concerning for seniors. Nutrition can play a role in preventing these illnesses:

1. Vitamin C: Consuming foods rich in vitamin C, like citrus fruits, strawberries, and bell peppers, may reduce the risk of respiratory infections.

2. Zinc: Zinc supports the immune system and may help prevent respiratory illnesses. Sources include lean meats, beans, and nuts.

3. Fluids: Staying well-hydrated with water and warm beverages can soothe the respiratory tract and thin mucus.

4. Garlic: Garlic contains compounds with antimicrobial properties and may help protect against respiratory infections.

5. Proactive Vaccination: Consult your healthcare provider about recommended vaccinations to prevent specific respiratory illnesses.

Lifestyle Choices for Immune Health

Nutrition is just one component of immune support. Consider these lifestyle choices for overall well-being:

1. Adequate Sleep: Prioritize quality sleep, as it is essential for immune function and overall health.

2. Stress Management: Chronic stress can weaken the immune system. Engage in relaxation techniques, such as meditation or yoga.

3. Physical Activity: Regular exercise supports immune function and overall vitality.

4. Avoid Smoking: Smoking can compromise immune health. Seek support to quit smoking if needed.

5. Social Interaction: Maintain social connections, as they contribute to mental and emotional well-being.

Proactive nutrition is a valuable tool in guarding against common ailments that can impact seniors. By focusing on immune-boosting foods, staying well-hydrated, and adopting a healthy lifestyle, you can enhance your resilience and enjoy a more vibrant and illness-free senior life.

4.7 Cancer Prevention: Dietary Strategies for Reducing Risk

Cancer prevention becomes increasingly important as you age, and nutrition can play a vital role in reducing the risk of developing various types of cancer. In this section, we'll explore dietary strategies and cancer-fighting foods to help you reduce your cancer risk and maintain optimal well-being.

Understanding the Role of Nutrition in Cancer Prevention

The relationship between diet and cancer risk is complex, but several dietary factors can influence your susceptibility to cancer. Here are key considerations:

1. Antioxidants: Antioxidants found in fruits and vegetables, such as vitamins C and E, selenium, and beta-carotene, can help neutralize free radicals and protect cells from DNA damage.

2. Fiber: Dietary fiber from whole grains, fruits, and vegetables may reduce the risk of colorectal cancer and promote digestive health.

3. Cruciferous Vegetables: Vegetables like broccoli, cauliflower, and Brussels sprouts contain compounds that may help prevent certain types of cancer.

4. Lean Proteins: Choosing lean protein sources like poultry, fish, and legumes can be part of a cancer-preventive diet.

5. Hydration: Staying well-hydrated with water is essential for overall health, including cancer prevention.

Dietary Strategies for Cancer Prevention

While no single food can prevent cancer, adopting a balanced and plant-rich diet can contribute to reducing your risk. Consider these dietary strategies:

1. Eat a Rainbow: Consume a wide variety of colorful fruits and vegetables daily to maximize your intake of vitamins, minerals, and antioxidants.

2. Whole Grains: Opt for whole grains like brown rice, quinoa, and whole wheat bread, which provide fiber and nutrients.

3. Limit Processed Meats: Reduce consumption of processed meats like bacon, hot dogs, and deli meats, as they are associated with an increased risk of colorectal cancer.

4. Healthy Fats: Incorporate healthy fats from sources like avocados, nuts, seeds, and olive oil while minimizing saturated and trans fats.

5. Alcohol in Moderation: If you consume alcohol, do so in moderation. Excessive alcohol intake is linked to several types of cancer.

6. Weight Management: Maintain a healthy weight through balanced eating and regular physical activity, as excess body weight is a risk factor for several cancers.

7. Stay Active: Engage in regular physical activity to support overall well-being and reduce cancer risk.

8. Food Preparation: Use healthy cooking methods like grilling, steaming, and roasting, and avoid charred or burnt foods, which may contain carcinogens.

Specific Foods with Cancer-Fighting Properties

While no specific food guarantees cancer prevention, some have shown promising properties in reducing cancer risk:

- **Berries:** Rich in antioxidants and phytochemicals, berries like blueberries, strawberries, and raspberries may help protect against cancer.

- **Tomatoes:** Tomatoes contain lycopene, a compound associated with a reduced risk of prostate cancer.

- **Leafy Greens:** Leafy greens like kale, spinach, and Swiss chard provide vitamins and minerals linked to cancer prevention.

- **Garlic:** Garlic contains sulfur compounds that may have anticancer effects.

- **Green Tea:** Green tea is rich in antioxidants called catechins, which may reduce the risk of certain cancers.

Cancer prevention is a lifelong commitment to healthy eating and lifestyle choices. By incorporating cancer-fighting foods and dietary practices into your daily life, you can proactively reduce your risk of developing cancer and support your overall well-being.

4.8 Digestive Health: Nourishing a Happy Gut

Maintaining digestive health is essential for seniors to enjoy comfortable and nourishing meals. In this section, we'll delve into the intricacies of digestive health, exploring dietary strategies and gut-friendly foods that can help you maintain optimal digestive function and overall well-being.

Understanding Digestive Health for Seniors

Digestive health is central to the absorption of nutrients and the elimination of waste from the body. Aging can bring about changes in digestive function, but there are steps you can take to support your digestive system:

1. Fiber Intake: Dietary fiber is crucial for regular bowel movements and overall digestive health. Include high-fiber foods like whole grains, fruits, vegetables, and legumes in your diet.

2. Hydration: Proper hydration with water helps soften stool and prevent constipation.

3. Probiotics: Probiotics are beneficial bacteria that support a healthy gut microbiome. Foods like yogurt, kefir, sauerkraut, and kimchi contain probiotics.

4. Prebiotics: Prebiotics are dietary fibers that nourish beneficial gut bacteria. They can be found in foods like garlic, onions, leeks, and asparagus.

5. Portion Control: Overeating can strain the digestive system. Pay attention to portion sizes to avoid discomfort.

6. Physical Activity: Regular physical activity can promote healthy digestion by encouraging regular bowel movements.

7. Food Tolerance: As you age, you may develop food intolerances. Pay attention to how your body reacts to specific foods and make adjustments as needed.

Dietary Strategies for Digestive Health

Adopting a digestive-friendly diet involves making choices that promote comfortable digestion and prevent common digestive issues. Consider these strategies:

1. Balanced Meals: Aim for balanced meals that include fiber-rich foods, lean proteins, healthy fats, and a variety of fruits and vegetables.

2. High-Fiber Foods: Include plenty of high-fiber foods in your diet to support regular bowel movements and prevent constipation.

3. Probiotic Foods: Incorporate probiotic-rich foods like yogurt, kefir, and fermented vegetables to promote a healthy gut microbiome.

4. Hydration: Drink adequate water throughout the day to keep your digestive system functioning smoothly.

5. Mindful Eating: Practice mindful eating to savor your meals, aid digestion, and prevent overeating.

6. Food Diary: Keeping a food diary can help you identify specific foods that may trigger digestive discomfort or intolerance.

7. Whole Foods: Choose whole, unprocessed foods over highly processed options, as they are generally gentler on the digestive system.

Foods for Digestive Comfort

Certain foods are known for their digestive benefits:

- **Ginger:** Ginger can help alleviate nausea and support digestion.

- **Bananas:** Bananas are gentle on the stomach and can help soothe digestive discomfort.

- **Papaya:** Papaya contains an enzyme called papain, which aids in digestion.

- **Peppermint:** Peppermint tea or peppermint oil may ease digestive symptoms like gas and bloating.

Nourishing a happy gut is essential for senior well-being. By incorporating digestive-friendly foods and dietary practices into your daily life, you can support optimal digestive function and enjoy comfortable and satisfying meals.

4.9 Nutritional Support for Common Medications

Many seniors rely on medications to manage various health conditions. Nutrition can play a crucial role in supporting the effectiveness of these medications and minimizing potential side effects. In this section, we'll explore how dietary choices can complement common medications and contribute to overall well-being.

Understanding the Medication-Nutrition Connection

Certain medications may interact with specific nutrients or dietary components, affecting their absorption, effectiveness, or side effects. It's essential to be aware of these interactions and make informed dietary choices:

1. **Anticoagulants:** Blood-thinning medications like warfarin (Coumadin) may require consistent vitamin K intake. Leafy greens like kale and spinach are rich in vitamin K, so maintaining a consistent intake can help with medication management.

2. **Statins:** Statins are prescribed to lower cholesterol levels. Coenzyme Q10 (CoQ10) supplements may be recommended alongside statins, as these medications can deplete CoQ10 levels in the body.

3. **Bone Health Medications:** Some medications prescribed for osteoporosis may require specific dietary instructions, such as taking them on an empty stomach or with a full glass of water.

4. **Diuretics:** Diuretics, which promote urination, can lead to potassium loss. Eating potassium-rich foods like bananas, oranges, and sweet potatoes can help maintain healthy potassium levels.

5. Acid-Suppressing Medications: Proton pump inhibitors (PPIs) and H2 blockers can reduce stomach acid, potentially affecting the absorption of certain nutrients like vitamin B12, calcium, and magnesium. Discuss potential supplementation with your healthcare provider.

6. Antibiotics: Antibiotics can disrupt the balance of beneficial gut bacteria. Consuming probiotic-rich foods or supplements can help restore gut health during and after antibiotic treatment.

7. Interaction with Food: Some medications should be taken with food to minimize gastrointestinal side effects, while others should be taken on an empty stomach for optimal absorption. Follow your healthcare provider's instructions regarding food and medication timing.

Nutritional Strategies to Support Medications

To maximize the benefits of your medications and minimize potential complications, consider these nutritional strategies:

1. Consult Your Healthcare Provider: Always communicate with your healthcare provider about your medications and any dietary concerns or potential interactions.

2. Consistent Intake: Maintain a consistent dietary routine to ensure medications are taken as directed and to minimize variability in nutrient intake.

3. Balanced Diet: Aim for a balanced diet rich in a variety of nutrients to support overall health and well-being.

4. Monitor Nutrient Levels: If you are on long-term medication, consider regular monitoring of relevant nutrient levels through blood tests to catch deficiencies early.

5. Consider Supplements: If nutrient deficiencies are identified, your healthcare provider may recommend supplements to address specific needs.

Nutritional support is a valuable component of medication management for seniors. By being aware of potential interactions, making informed dietary choices, and collaborating with healthcare providers, you can enhance the effectiveness of your medications and promote overall well-being.

5. PRACTICAL STEPS FOR SENIOR NUTRITION

Embracing senior nutrition isn't just about theory; it's about practical steps that lead to a healthier and more fulfilling life. In this section, we'll provide actionable advice and guidelines to help you navigate the world of nutrition and make informed choices that support your well-being.

1. Create a Balanced Plate

Start with a simple rule of thumb for every meal: aim for a balanced plate. Divide your plate into sections:

- **Half of Your Plate:** Fill it with colorful fruits and vegetables. These provide essential vitamins, minerals, and antioxidants.

- **One-Quarter of Your Plate:** Include a lean protein source like fish, poultry, beans, or tofu. Protein is vital for maintaining muscle mass.

- **One-Quarter of Your Plate:** Choose whole grains like brown rice, quinoa, or whole wheat pasta. They provide energy and fiber.

2. Pay Attention to Portions

As you age, your calorie needs may decrease, but the need for nutrients remains. Be mindful of portion sizes to avoid overeating. Use smaller plates and listen to your body's hunger and fullness cues.

3. Stay Hydrated

Dehydration can be more common in seniors and can lead to various health issues. Drink plenty of water throughout the day. Herbal teas and water-rich fruits like watermelon can also contribute to hydration.

4. Embrace Variety

Eating a wide variety of foods ensures you get a diverse range of nutrients. Don't be afraid to try new foods and recipes. Explore different cuisines to keep your meals exciting and nutritious.

5. Limit Processed Foods

Processed foods often contain excess salt, sugar, and unhealthy fats. Minimize your intake of processed snacks, sugary beverages, and fast food. Opt for whole, unprocessed foods whenever possible.

6. Practice Mindful Eating

Savor your meals. Eating mindfully means paying attention to the flavors, textures, and sensations of each bite. This can help prevent overeating and improve your relationship with food.

7. Consider Special Dietary Needs

If you have specific dietary needs or restrictions due to health conditions, consult with a registered dietitian or healthcare provider for personalized guidance.

8. Enjoy Social Eating

Share meals with friends and family whenever possible. Social interactions during meals can enhance your enjoyment of food and contribute to mental and emotional well-being.

9. Plan Ahead

Planning your meals and snacks can help you make healthier choices and avoid impulsive, less nutritious options. Prepare balanced meals in advance, and have healthy snacks readily available.

10. Be Mindful of Medications

If you're taking medications, be aware of any dietary interactions or instructions provided by your healthcare provider. Follow their advice regarding food and medication timing.

11. Stay Active

Physical activity complements good nutrition. Engage in regular exercise to support overall well-being and maintain muscle mass and strength.

12. Seek Support

Don't hesitate to seek support from a registered dietitian or nutritionist if you have specific dietary concerns or health conditions that require personalized guidance.

Practical steps for senior nutrition involve not only what you eat but how you approach food. By following these guidelines, you can make informed dietary choices that promote a healthier and more vibrant senior life. Remember that nutrition is an ongoing journey, and small, sustainable changes can have a significant impact on your well-being.

5.1. Creating a Senior-Friendly Kitchen

Your kitchen is the heart of your nutritional journey, and making it senior-friendly can greatly enhance your cooking experience and meal preparation. In this section, we'll explore practical steps to create a kitchen that promotes safe and enjoyable cooking for seniors.

1. Organize for Accessibility

Arrange your kitchen so that frequently used items are easily accessible. This includes pots, pans, utensils, and ingredients. Store these items at waist height or lower to avoid stretching or reaching.

2. Install Proper Lighting

Good lighting is essential for safe cooking. Ensure your kitchen is well-lit, especially in work areas like countertops and stovetops. Consider under-cabinet lighting to brighten workspaces.

3. Non-Slip Flooring

Choose flooring that is slip-resistant to prevent accidents. Mats with non-slip backing in front of the sink or stove can add an extra layer of safety.

4. Easy-to-Use Appliances

Opt for kitchen appliances with user-friendly features. Look for appliances with large, easy-to-read buttons and controls. Appliances with automatic shut-off functions provide an added layer of safety.

5. Adequate Seating

Include a comfortable chair or stool in the kitchen for breaks during meal preparation. Having a place to sit can reduce fatigue and make cooking more enjoyable.

6. Kitchen Tools

Invest in ergonomic kitchen tools that are easy to grip and use. Tools with large, comfortable handles can reduce strain on the hands and wrists.

7. Clear Countertops

Keep countertops clear of clutter to create a spacious and safe workspace. This also makes it easier to clean up spills promptly.

8. Safe Cooking Surfaces

Ensure your stovetop and oven are in good working condition. If necessary, consider installing safety features like automatic shut-off timers.

9. Accessibility Aids

Install grab bars or handrails near high-risk areas like the stove or sink to provide extra support and stability.

10. Fire Safety

Place a fire extinguisher in an easily accessible location in case of kitchen fires. Review fire safety procedures regularly.

11. Kitchen Layout

If possible, arrange your kitchen so that the stove, sink, and refrigerator are in a convenient triangle layout. This minimizes excessive movement during meal preparation.

12. Shelf and Cabinet Organization

Use pull-out or pull-down shelves and cabinets to make reaching items in higher spaces more manageable. Lazy Susans or rotating shelves can also improve accessibility.

13. Meal Prep Aids

Consider pre-cut vegetables, pre-cooked grains, and other convenience items to simplify meal preparation.

14. Anti-Scald Devices

Install anti-scald devices on faucets to prevent accidental burns from hot water.

15. Regular Maintenance

Regularly inspect and maintain your kitchen appliances and fixtures to ensure they are in good working condition.

Creating a senior-friendly kitchen is a practical step towards promoting safe and enjoyable cooking experiences. By implementing these adjustments and ensuring that your kitchen is both functional and comfortable, you can continue to prepare nutritious meals with ease and confidence.

5.2. Setting Up a Nutrient-Focused Kitchen

Transforming your kitchen into a nutrient-focused hub is a powerful way to support your journey toward better health through nutrition. In this section, we'll explore practical steps to set up a kitchen that encourages the selection and preparation of nutrient-dense meals.

1. Stock Up on Nutrient-Rich Foods

Fill your pantry, refrigerator, and freezer with a variety of nutrient-rich foods. These should include:

- **Whole Grains:** Such as brown rice, quinoa, whole wheat pasta, and oats.

- **Fruits and Vegetables:** Fresh, frozen, or canned (preferably without added sugar or salt).

- **Lean Proteins:** Such as poultry, fish, lean cuts of beef or pork, tofu, and legumes.

- **Healthy Fats:** Including olive oil, avocados, nuts, and seeds.

- **Low-Fat Dairy or Dairy Alternatives:** Choose options with minimal added sugars.

- **Herbs and Spices:** To add flavor without excess salt or sugar.

2. Meal Planning Tools

Invest in meal planning tools like a whiteboard or chalkboard to schedule meals and create shopping lists. This helps you stay organized and ensures you have the ingredients needed for nutritious meals.

3. Portion Control

Use measuring cups, spoons, and a kitchen scale to help control portion sizes. This is especially important for seniors to avoid overeating.

4. Food Storage Containers

Invest in a variety of food storage containers to store leftovers and prepped ingredients. Transparent containers make it easy to see what's inside and reduce food waste.

5. Nutrition Labels

Learn how to read nutrition labels to make informed choices when purchasing packaged foods. Pay attention to serving sizes, calories, and nutrient content.

6. Food Processor or Blender

A food processor or blender can be invaluable for creating nutrient-packed smoothies, purees, and sauces using fruits, vegetables, and healthy fats.

7. Kitchen Gadgets

Consider gadgets like a spiralizer for turning vegetables into healthy "noodles," a steamer for preserving nutrients during cooking, and a salad spinner for easy salad preparation.

8. Spice Rack

A well-stocked spice rack can add flavor to your meals without the need for excessive salt or sugar. Include options like cinnamon, turmeric, cumin, and paprika.

9. Nutrient-Dense Snacks

Keep nutrient-dense snacks on hand for convenient and healthy munching. Examples include unsalted nuts, Greek yogurt, and cut-up vegetables.

10. Meal Prep Containers

Invest in containers designed for meal prepping. These can help you portion out meals and snacks in advance, making it easier to stick to a nutrient-focused eating plan.

11. Water Filtration

Consider a water filtration system to ensure you have access to clean, fresh water for hydration and cooking.

12. Spice Up Your Meals

Experiment with new herbs and spices to add variety and flavor to your dishes. This can make nutrient-dense meals more enjoyable.

A nutrient-focused kitchen sets the stage for healthier eating habits. By stocking up on nutrient-rich foods, equipping your kitchen with the right tools, and emphasizing portion control and meal planning, you can create an environment that supports your journey to improved health and well-being through nutrition.

Equipping your kitchen with the right tools and adopting smart cooking techniques can simplify meal preparation and enhance your culinary adventures. In this section, we'll explore essential kitchen tools and share tips to make your cooking experience more enjoyable and efficient.

Essential Kitchen Tools for Seniors

1. **Quality Knives:** Invest in sharp, high-quality knives for slicing, dicing, and chopping. Keeping them sharp ensures safer and more efficient cutting.

2. **Cutting Boards:** Use cutting boards made of materials like wood or plastic. Consider color-coding boards to prevent cross-contamination when handling different foods.

3. **Non-Slip Mats:** Place non-slip mats beneath your cutting board and mixing bowls to keep them stable during meal preparation.

4. **Pots and Pans:** Opt for non-stick pots and pans to reduce the need for excessive oil or butter when cooking.

5. **Food Processor:** A food processor can help with chopping, shredding, and mixing ingredients for various recipes.

6. **Blender:** A blender is excellent for making smoothies, soups, and sauces using fruits, vegetables, and healthy fats.

7. **Microwave Oven:** Microwave ovens are handy for reheating leftovers and cooking certain foods quickly.

8. **Slow Cooker:** Slow cookers or crockpots are perfect for preparing easy, one-pot meals that require minimal effort.

9. **Toaster Oven:** Toaster ovens are versatile appliances for toasting, baking, and broiling small portions of food.

10. **Measuring Cups and Spoons:** Accurate measurement is crucial for portion control and consistent results.

11. **Can Opener:** Choose a user-friendly can opener that doesn't require excessive strength to operate.

12. **Mixing Bowls:** Have a variety of mixing bowls in different sizes for blending and preparing ingredients.

Smart Cooking Tips for Seniors

1. **Prep in Advance:** Take advantage of times when you have energy to prepare ingredients or even full meals. This makes cooking on busier days more manageable.

2. **Frozen Fruits and Vegetables:** Keep a stock of frozen fruits and vegetables on hand for convenience. They retain their nutrients and are easy to incorporate into meals.

3. **One-Pot Meals:** Explore one-pot recipes that simplify cooking and minimize cleanup. These can be particularly helpful for seniors.

4. **Batch Cooking:** Prepare larger quantities of meals and freeze individual portions for future use. This saves time and ensures nutritious options are readily available.

5. **Meal Delivery Services:** Consider meal delivery services that offer healthy, pre-prepared meals if cooking becomes challenging.

6. **Slow Cooking:** Utilize a slow cooker for effortless meal preparation. Simply add ingredients, set it, and return to a delicious meal.

7. **Double Recipes:** When you do cook, consider doubling the recipe to have leftovers for the next day or for freezing.

8. **Kitchen Safety:** Pay attention to kitchen safety, including using oven mitts, avoiding slippery floors, and having a fire extinguisher on hand.

9. **Adapted Utensils:** If you have dexterity challenges, explore adapted utensils designed for easier use.

10. **Enjoy the Process:** Cooking can be an enjoyable and creative activity. Savor the experience, and don't be afraid to try new recipes and flavors.

Equipping your kitchen with the right tools and adopting smart cooking practices can make meal preparation enjoyable and manageable for seniors. Whether you're looking to simplify your cooking routine or explore new culinary horizons, these tools and tips can enhance your experience in the kitchen.

5.4. Meal Planning and Preparation

Effective meal planning and preparation are keys to maintaining a healthy and balanced diet. In this section, we'll explore the importance of meal planning and share practical tips to make meal preparation more efficient and enjoyable.

The Importance of Meal Planning

Meal planning offers numerous benefits for seniors:

1. **Nutritional Balance:** Planning meals in advance allows you to ensure that each meal includes a variety of nutrient-rich foods.

2. **Portion Control:** You can manage portion sizes more effectively, preventing overeating.

3. **Budgeting:** Meal planning can help you budget your grocery expenses and reduce food waste.

4. **Convenience:** Having meals and snacks ready to go saves time and energy, especially on busy days.

5. **Nutrient Focus:** It enables you to create nutrient-dense meals tailored to your specific health needs.

Practical Meal Planning Tips

1. **Set a Schedule:** Establish regular meal times to create a routine. Consistency can improve digestion and metabolism.

2. **Plan Your Week:** Take time each week to plan your meals and snacks. Consider your schedule and choose recipes that suit your available time and energy.

3. **Use a Planner:** Invest in a meal planner or use a digital tool or app to organize your meal plans and shopping lists.

4. **Include Variety:** Ensure your meal plan includes a variety of food groups and colors. Different foods offer different nutrients.

5. **Shop with a List:** Stick to your grocery list to avoid impulse purchases. This can save you money and reduce food waste.

6. **Prep Ingredients:** Wash, chop, and portion out ingredients in advance to make cooking quicker and more enjoyable.

7. **Batch Cooking:** Cook larger quantities and freeze individual portions for future meals. This is especially helpful when you don't feel like cooking.

8. **Explore New Recipes:** Keep things interesting by trying new recipes or cuisines. Experiment with different flavors and ingredients.

Efficient Meal Preparation

1. **One-Pot Meals:** Choose recipes that require minimal dishes and cooking steps. One-pot meals simplify cleanup.

2. **Crockpot Convenience:** Utilize a slow cooker for effortless meal preparation. Set it in the morning, and return to a ready meal.

3. **Pre-Chop Ingredients:** Purchase pre-chopped or frozen fruits and vegetables to save time. Pre-cutting ingredients when you have energy can also help.

4. **Multi-Tasking:** When possible, prepare multiple components of a meal simultaneously to save time.

5. **Leftovers:** Plan for leftovers and enjoy them for lunch or dinner the next day. Many dishes taste even better after flavors meld.

6. **Cook in Batches:** Cook grains like rice or quinoa in larger batches and use them in various meals throughout the week.

Meal planning and preparation are essential tools for maintaining a nutritious and satisfying diet as a senior. By incorporating these practices into your routine and tailoring them to your needs, you can make eating well a seamless part of your daily life.

5.5. Monthly Meal Plans for a Year of Health

5.6. Seasonal Recipes and Meal Planning

Eating with the seasons not only provides variety but also ensures that you enjoy the freshest and most flavorful ingredients. In this section, we'll explore the benefits of seasonal eating and provide recipes and meal planning tips for each season of the year.

Spring

Benefits of Spring Eating:

- Fresh and vibrant produce.

- Lighter and refreshing meals.

- Opportunity to detoxify with greens.

Sample Spring Meal Plan:

Week 1:

- **Breakfast:** Strawberry and spinach smoothie.

- **Lunch:** Grilled asparagus and quinoa salad.

- **Dinner:** Lemon herb roasted chicken with steamed broccoli.

Week 2:

- **Breakfast:** Greek yogurt parfait with mixed berries.

- **Lunch:** Spring pea soup with a side of whole grain bread.

- **Dinner:** Baked salmon with dill sauce and roasted carrots.

Week 3:

- **Breakfast:** Scrambled eggs with fresh chives and whole wheat toast.

- **Lunch:** Spinach and strawberry salad with grilled chicken.

- **Dinner:** Veggie-packed stir-fried tofu with brown rice.

Week 4:

- **Breakfast:** Rhubarb and yogurt parfait.

- **Lunch:** Spinach and feta stuffed bell peppers.

- **Dinner:** Herb-crusted tilapia with sautéed asparagus.

Summer

Benefits of Summer Eating:

- Abundance of fruits and vegetables.

- Ideal for light, outdoor dining.

- Perfect for salads, grilling, and fresh herbs.

Sample Summer Meal Plan:

Week 1:

- **Breakfast:** Watermelon and mint smoothie.

- **Lunch:** Caprese salad with ripe tomatoes, mozzarella, and basil.

- **Dinner:** Grilled shrimp skewers with a Mediterranean quinoa salad.

Week 2:

- **Breakfast:** Yogurt parfait with fresh berries and granola.

- **Lunch:** Cucumber and dill Greek yogurt dip with veggie sticks.

- **Dinner:** BBQ chicken with coleslaw and corn on the cob.

Week 3:

- **Breakfast:** Peach and almond milk overnight oats.

- **Lunch:** Spinach and watermelon salad with feta and balsamic vinaigrette.

- **Dinner:** Grilled vegetable platter with herb-marinated chicken.

Week 4:

- **Breakfast:** Kiwi and banana smoothie bowl.

- **Lunch:** Chilled gazpacho soup with a side of whole grain crackers.

- **Dinner:** Lemon-herb grilled trout with quinoa and steamed green beans.

Autumn

Benefits of Autumn Eating:

- Harvest of root vegetables and hearty greens.

- Perfect for warming soups and stews.

- Ideal for cozy and comforting dishes.

Sample Autumn Meal Plan:

Week 1:

- **Breakfast:** Apple cinnamon oatmeal.

- **Lunch:** Butternut squash and apple soup with a side salad.

- **Dinner:** Roast turkey with cranberry sauce and roasted Brussels sprouts.

Week 2:

- **Breakfast:** Pumpkin spice yogurt parfait.

- **Lunch:** Sweet potato and black bean chili.

- **Dinner:** Maple-glazed salmon with roasted acorn squash and quinoa.

Week 3:

- **Breakfast:** Spiced pear and walnut smoothie.

- **Lunch:** Kale and quinoa salad with roasted root vegetables.

- **Dinner:** Beef stew with hearty vegetables.

Week 4:

- **Breakfast:** Baked apple oatmeal.

- **Lunch:** Creamy mushroom and barley soup.

- **Dinner:** Herb-crusted pork chops with mashed sweet potatoes and green beans.

Winter

Benefits of Winter Eating:

- Comforting and warming meals.

- Opportunity for slow-cooked dishes.

- Access to citrus fruits for vitamin C.

Sample Winter Meal Plan:

Week 1:

- **Breakfast:** Citrus and yogurt parfait.

- **Lunch:** Chicken and vegetable noodle soup.

- **Dinner:** Baked cod with lemon and garlic, served with quinoa and steamed broccoli.

Week 2:

- **Breakfast:** Banana and walnut baked oatmeal.

- **Lunch:** Spinach and mandarin orange salad with grilled chicken.

- **Dinner:** Beef and vegetable stir-fry with brown rice.

Week 3:

- **Breakfast:** Cranberry and almond smoothie.

- **Lunch:** Lentil and vegetable stew.

- **Dinner:** Herb-roasted turkey breast with roasted Brussels sprouts and sweet potato.

Week 4:

- **Breakfast:** Spiced pear and pecan oatmeal.

- **Lunch:** Creamy potato and leek soup.

- **Dinner:** Baked salmon with a honey-mustard glaze, served with quinoa and steamed asparagus.

Eating seasonally not only supports your health but also connects you to the natural rhythms of the year. By incorporating fresh, seasonal ingredients into your meal plans, you can enjoy the flavors of each season while nourishing your body with diverse nutrients.

CHAPTER 6: DELICIOUS AND NUTRITIOUS RECIPES FOR SENIORS

In this chapter, we delve into a treasure trove of mouthwatering and health-enhancing recipes specially curated for seniors. Each recipe is designed to not only tantalize your taste buds but also provide the essential nutrients your body needs for vitality and well-being. These recipes are easy to prepare and packed with flavor, ensuring that your journey to better health is both enjoyable and satisfying.

6.1 Meal Plans for Seniors

Week 1:

Day 1:

- **Breakfast:** Scrambled eggs with spinach and whole-grain toast.

- **Lunch:** Turkey and avocado wrap with a side of mixed greens.

- **Dinner:** Baked salmon with quinoa and steamed broccoli.

Day 2:

- **Breakfast:** Oatmeal with sliced bananas and chopped walnuts.

- **Lunch:** Chickpea salad with cucumbers, tomatoes, and a lemon-tahini dressing.

- **Dinner:** Grilled chicken breast with sweet potato and green beans.

Day 3:

- **Breakfast:** Greek yogurt parfait with mixed berries and honey.

- **Lunch:** Spinach and feta stuffed bell peppers with a side salad.

- **Dinner:** Lentil soup with whole-grain bread.

Day 4:

- **Breakfast:** Smoothie with kale, pineapple, almond milk, and protein powder.

- **Lunch:** Quinoa and black bean salad with a lime-cilantro dressing.

- **Dinner:** Baked cod with lemon and dill, served with quinoa and steamed asparagus.

Day 5:

- **Breakfast:** Scrambled eggs with sautéed mushrooms and whole-grain toast.

- **Lunch:** Caprese salad with mozzarella, tomatoes, and basil.

- **Dinner:** Beef and broccoli stir-fry with brown rice.

Day 6:

- **Breakfast:** Overnight oats with chia seeds, almond milk, and mixed berries.

- **Lunch:** Spinach and walnut salad with grilled chicken and balsamic vinaigrette.

- **Dinner:** Grilled shrimp with brown rice and steamed broccoli.

Day 7:

- **Breakfast:** Whole-grain waffles with mixed fruit compote and Greek yogurt.

- **Lunch:** Spinach and strawberry salad with grilled chicken.

- **Dinner:** Herb-roasted turkey breast with roasted Brussels sprouts and quinoa.

Weeks 2-4: Repeat the meal plan for weeks 2, 3, and 4 to complete the month. You can make adjustments by swapping out specific ingredients, incorporating seasonal produce, and introducing new recipes to keep the meals interesting.

Remember that individual dietary needs may vary, so it's essential to consult with a healthcare provider or registered dietitian to create a personalized meal plan that considers any specific health conditions, allergies, or dietary restrictions for the senior in question.

6.2 Seasonal Recipes for Seniors

Spring Recipe: Asparagus and Salmon Salad

Ingredients:

- 6-8 asparagus spears, trimmed

- 4 oz baked or grilled salmon, flaked

- Mixed greens or spinach

- Cherry tomatoes, halved

- 1/4 cup sliced almonds, toasted

- Lemon-tahini dressing (lemon juice, tahini, olive oil, garlic, salt, and pepper)

Instructions:

1. Steam the asparagus until tender-crisp, then plunge them into ice water to stop cooking.

2. Arrange the mixed greens on a plate, top with asparagus, flaked salmon, cherry tomatoes, and toasted almonds.

3. Drizzle with lemon-tahini dressing.

Summer Recipe: Caprese Stuffed Avocado

Ingredients:

- 2 ripe avocados, halved and pitted

- 1 cup cherry tomatoes, halved

- Fresh mozzarella cheese, diced

- Fresh basil leaves

- Balsamic glaze

- Olive oil

- Salt and pepper to taste

Instructions:

1. Scoop out a bit of flesh from each avocado half to create a small well.

2. In a bowl, combine cherry tomatoes, diced mozzarella, and torn basil leaves. Drizzle with olive oil, season with salt and pepper.

3. Fill each avocado half with the tomato-mozzarella-basil mixture.

4. Drizzle with balsamic glaze before serving.

Autumn Recipe: Butternut Squash Soup

Ingredients:

- 1 medium butternut squash, peeled, seeded, and diced

- 1 onion, diced

- 2 carrots, peeled and chopped

- 2 apples, peeled, cored, and chopped

- 4 cups vegetable broth

- 1 tsp ground cinnamon

- 1/2 tsp ground nutmeg

- Salt and pepper to taste

- Olive oil

Instructions:

1. In a large pot, sauté diced onion and carrots in olive oil until softened.

2. Add the diced butternut squash and apples, and cook for a few minutes.

3. Pour in the vegetable broth, add ground cinnamon and nutmeg. Season with salt and pepper.

4. Bring to a boil, then reduce heat, cover, and simmer until the vegetables are tender.

5. Use an immersion blender to puree the soup until smooth.

6. Serve with a sprinkle of nutmeg and a dollop of Greek yogurt if desired.

Winter Recipe: Herb-Crusted Roast Chicken

Ingredients:

- 4 boneless, skinless chicken breasts

- 2 tsp dried thyme

- 2 tsp dried rosemary

- 1 tsp garlic powder

- Salt and pepper to taste

- Olive oil

Instructions:

1. Preheat the oven to 375°F (190°C).

2. In a bowl, combine dried thyme, dried rosemary, garlic powder, salt, and pepper.

3. Brush chicken breasts with olive oil and sprinkle the herb mixture evenly over them.

4. Place the chicken on a baking sheet and roast in the oven until cooked through (about 25-30 minutes).

5. Serve with your choice of steamed vegetables and a side of quinoa or brown rice.

These seasonal recipes can provide delicious and nutritious options for seniors throughout the year. Don't forget to consider any specific dietary

CHAPTER 7: ACHIEVING LONGEVITY THROUGH NUTRITION

In this chapter, we delve into the profound connection between nutrition and longevity. Longevity is not merely about adding years to your life but ensuring that those years are filled with vitality, good health, and a high quality of life. The choices you make in your diet play a pivotal role in achieving this goal.

As a senior, your nutritional needs may evolve, and understanding how to nourish your body optimally becomes even more crucial. The good news is that with the right knowledge and approach, you can enhance your longevity and enjoy the benefits of a well-balanced and nourishing diet.

In this chapter, we will explore:

7.1. The Link Between Nutrition and Longevity: Discover how the foods you consume impact the aging process and influence your overall health.

7.2. Antioxidants and Aging: Explore the role of antioxidants in combating oxidative stress and promoting longevity.

7.3. Superfoods for a Long Life: Learn about specific foods that are celebrated for their potential to support longevity.

7.4. Mindful Eating for a Longer Life: Explore the concept of mindful eating and how it can contribute to healthier eating habits.

7.5. Hydration and Longevity: Understand the importance of staying well-hydrated for overall well-being.

7.6. Staying Active in Your Senior Years: Discover the synergy between nutrition and physical activity for a longer and healthier life.

7.7. Emotional Well-Being and Longevity: Learn about the connection between emotional health, stress management, and longevity.

7.8. The Role of Social Connections: Explore how maintaining social connections can positively impact your longevity.

As you delve into the pages of this chapter, you'll gain insights into the principles of longevity through nutrition and lifestyle choices. These insights will empower you to make informed decisions about your diet and overall well-being, setting the stage for a longer, healthier, and more vibrant life.

7.1. The Link Between Nutrition and Longevity

Nutrition and longevity share an intricate relationship that can significantly impact the aging process and overall quality of life for seniors. The choices you make regarding your diet have a profound influence on your ability to live a longer, healthier, and more fulfilling life.

Understanding the Key Connections:

1. **Cellular Health:** Proper nutrition supports the health of your cells. This is crucial because aging involves the natural breakdown of cells over time. A diet rich in antioxidants, vitamins, and minerals can help mitigate cell damage caused by oxidative stress, a primary contributor to aging.

2. **Inflammation Control:** Chronic inflammation is linked to a range of age-related diseases. Certain foods, such as fatty fish rich in omega-3 fatty acids, colorful fruits and vegetables, and whole grains, have anti-inflammatory properties and can reduce the risk of age-related inflammation.

3. **Heart Health:** Cardiovascular health is closely tied to longevity. A diet low in saturated fats and high in fiber, particularly from whole grains, fruits, and vegetables, can support heart health and reduce the risk of heart disease.

4. **Brain Function:** Cognitive decline is a concern for many seniors. Nutrients like omega-3 fatty acids, antioxidants, and B vitamins found in foods like fatty fish, berries, and leafy greens can promote brain health and potentially delay cognitive decline.

5. **Bone Strength:** As you age, maintaining bone health becomes critical. Calcium and vitamin D from dairy products, fortified foods, and supplements when necessary, along with foods rich in

vitamin K like leafy greens, support bone strength and may prevent fractures.

6. **Gut Health:** The gut microbiome plays a role in overall health. A diet high in fiber from fruits, vegetables, and whole grains can promote a diverse and healthy gut microbiome, potentially reducing the risk of digestive issues and other health problems.

7. **Immune Function:** A well-balanced diet ensures that your immune system remains robust. Vitamins and minerals, particularly vitamin C, vitamin D, and zinc, support immune function, helping the body fight off illnesses and infections.

8. **Weight Management:** Maintaining a healthy weight is associated with longevity. A diet that provides the right balance of nutrients can help you manage your weight effectively.

In the pages that follow, we will delve deeper into these connections and explore specific nutrients and foods that can promote longevity. By understanding how nutrition affects your body at a cellular level, you can make informed choices to enhance your health and extend your years of vitality.

7.2. Antioxidants and Aging

Antioxidants are like the superheroes of the nutritional world when it comes to combating the effects of aging. These powerful compounds play a pivotal role in protecting your cells from oxidative stress, a key driver of aging and age-related diseases. Understanding the significance of antioxidants and incorporating them into your diet can be a game-changer for promoting longevity.

The Role of Antioxidants:

Oxidative stress occurs when there's an imbalance between free radicals and antioxidants in your body. Free radicals are unstable molecules that can damage cells, proteins, and DNA, contributing to the aging process and the development of chronic diseases. Antioxidants neutralize these harmful free radicals, reducing their potential damage.

Sources of Antioxidants:

1. **Vitamin C:** Found in citrus fruits, strawberries, bell peppers, and broccoli, vitamin C is a potent antioxidant that supports skin health and immune function.

2. **Vitamin E:** Nuts, seeds, and vegetable oils are rich sources of vitamin E, which helps protect cells from oxidative damage.

3. **Beta-Carotene:** This antioxidant is found in brightly colored fruits and vegetables like carrots, sweet potatoes, and spinach. It's converted into vitamin A in the body, which is crucial for eye health.

4. **Selenium:** Selenium is abundant in Brazil nuts, fish, and whole grains. It's a key player in the body's antioxidant defense system.

5. **Flavonoids:** These compounds are found in foods like berries, tea, and dark chocolate. They have anti-inflammatory and antioxidant properties.

6. **Polyphenols:** Present in foods such as red wine, green tea, and certain fruits, polyphenols have been associated with various health benefits, including antioxidant effects.

7. **Coenzyme Q10 (CoQ10):** CoQ10 is naturally produced in the body and is also found in foods like fish, meat, and whole grains. It helps protect cells from oxidative damage.

Incorporating Antioxidants into Your Diet:

To harness the power of antioxidants for aging gracefully, consider these dietary choices:

1. **Colorful Fruits and Vegetables:** Aim to fill your plate with a rainbow of fruits and vegetables, as different colors often indicate a variety of antioxidants.

2. **Healthy Fats:** Incorporate sources of healthy fats like nuts, seeds, and olive oil into your diet.

3. **Green Tea:** Enjoy a cup of green tea, rich in antioxidants, as a daily beverage.

4. **Berries:** Berries like blueberries, strawberries, and raspberries are antioxidant-packed superfoods.

5. **Nuts and Seeds:** Snack on a handful of nuts and seeds for a satisfying and antioxidant-rich treat.

6. **Whole Grains:** Opt for whole grains like brown rice, quinoa, and whole wheat, which provide essential nutrients and antioxidants.

By making these antioxidant-rich foods a regular part of your diet, you can help shield your cells from oxidative stress, potentially slowing down the aging process and promoting a longer, healthier life.

7.3. Superfoods for a Long Life

Superfoods are nutrient-dense foods that are celebrated for their exceptional health benefits. They are packed with vitamins, minerals, antioxidants, and other bioactive compounds that can support your quest for longevity. Including superfoods in your diet is like giving your body a potent dose of nourishment that can enhance your overall well-being.

Exploring Remarkable Superfoods:

1. **Blueberries:** These tiny powerhouses are rich in antioxidants, particularly anthocyanins, which have been linked to improved cognitive function and reduced oxidative stress.

2. **Leafy Greens:** Spinach, kale, Swiss chard, and collard greens are loaded with vitamins, minerals, and fiber. They support heart health, bone health, and provide essential nutrients.

3. **Salmon:** Fatty fish like salmon are abundant in omega-3 fatty acids, which promote heart health, reduce inflammation, and support brain function.

4. **Nuts and Seeds:** Almonds, walnuts, chia seeds, and flaxseeds are packed with healthy fats, fiber, and antioxidants. They can help lower cholesterol and reduce the risk of heart disease.

5. **Berries:** In addition to blueberries, strawberries, raspberries, and blackberries are rich in antioxidants, vitamins, and fiber, making them ideal for promoting overall health.

6. **Turmeric:** This spice contains curcumin, a potent anti-inflammatory compound. Turmeric has been associated with reduced inflammation and improved joint health.

7. **Greek Yogurt:** High in protein and probiotics, Greek yogurt supports gut health and provides essential nutrients like calcium and vitamin D for bone health.

8. **Broccoli:** This cruciferous vegetable is a nutritional powerhouse, supplying vitamins, fiber, and sulforaphane, a compound with potential cancer-fighting properties.

9. **Green Tea:** Known for its antioxidant content, green tea can support heart health, improve cognitive function, and may even aid in weight management.

10. **Avocado:** Rich in healthy fats, avocados provide heart-healthy monounsaturated fats, fiber, and essential nutrients.

Incorporating Superfoods into Your Diet:

To make the most of these superfoods, consider the following strategies:

- **Diversify Your Diet:** Aim to include a variety of superfoods in your meals to maximize their health benefits.

- **Smoothies:** Blend berries, spinach, Greek yogurt, and a touch of turmeric for a nutrient-packed morning smoothie.

- **Salads:** Create vibrant salads with leafy greens, nuts, seeds, and colorful vegetables.

- **Fish Dinners:** Enjoy fatty fish like salmon for dinner at least twice a week.

- **Healthy Snacks:** Keep a stash of nuts, seeds, and dried berries for quick, nutritious snacks.

- **Spice It Up:** Add turmeric and other spices to your dishes for both flavor and health benefits.

These superfoods can be key components of a diet aimed at promoting longevity. By incorporating them into your meals regularly, you provide your body with essential nutrients and antioxidants that can contribute to a longer and healthier life.

7.4. Mindful Eating for a Longer Life

Mindful eating is a practice that goes beyond the types of foods you consume; it's about how you consume them. This approach to eating can have a profound impact on your overall well-being and may contribute to a longer, healthier life.

The Essence of Mindful Eating:

Mindful eating is a concept rooted in mindfulness, a practice that encourages you to be fully present in the moment, paying close attention to your thoughts, feelings, and sensations. When applied to eating, mindful eating involves:

1. **Savoring Each Bite:** Instead of rushing through meals, take the time to appreciate the taste, texture, and aroma of your food. Engage your senses fully.

2. **Listening to Your Body:** Pay attention to your body's hunger and fullness cues. Eat when you're hungry and stop when you're satisfied, not when you're overly full.

3. **Eliminating Distractions:** Minimize distractions during meals. Turn off the TV, put away your phone, and focus solely on your food and the experience of eating.

4. **Eating with Intention:** Consider the nutritional value of the foods you choose. Opt for nourishing options that support your health and well-being.

Benefits of Mindful Eating:

Mindful eating can have a range of benefits that contribute to a longer life:

- **Weight Management:** By being attuned to your body's hunger and fullness cues, you're less likely to overeat, which can support weight management.

- **Digestive Health:** Eating slowly and mindfully can aid digestion and reduce digestive discomfort.

- **Reduced Stress:** Mindful eating can help reduce stress and emotional eating by promoting a sense of calm and awareness.

- **Improved Relationship with Food:** It fosters a healthier relationship with food, allowing you to enjoy meals without guilt or negative associations.

- **Enhanced Enjoyment:** When you savor each bite, you derive more pleasure from your food, making the dining experience more satisfying.

Practicing Mindful Eating:

To incorporate mindful eating into your daily life:

- Begin with small steps, like dedicating 5-10 minutes to eat without distractions.

- Use all your senses to engage with your food.

- Chew each bite thoroughly and savor the flavors.

- Pause between bites to assess your hunger and fullness.

- Be patient with yourself; mindful eating is a skill that develops over time.

By embracing mindful eating, you can transform your relationship with food and, in turn, enhance your overall well-being, potentially contributing to a longer and healthier life.

7.5. Hydration and Longevity

While it's often overlooked, proper hydration is a fundamental aspect of promoting longevity and maintaining overall health, especially for seniors. Water is not just a vital substance; it's the essence of life itself. Understanding the significance of hydration and adopting healthy drinking habits can significantly impact your well-being and contribute to a longer life.

The Role of Hydration:

Hydration is essential for numerous bodily functions, including:

1. **Cell Function:** Water is the medium in which cellular processes occur. Adequate hydration ensures that cells can function optimally.

2. **Temperature Regulation:** Proper hydration helps regulate body temperature, crucial for avoiding heat-related illnesses.

3. **Joint Health:** Staying hydrated lubricates joints, reducing the risk of joint pain and stiffness.

4. **Digestive Health:** Water aids in digestion, preventing constipation and supporting a healthy gut.

5. **Cognitive Function:** Dehydration can impair cognitive function, affecting memory and concentration.

6. **Detoxification:** Hydration supports the body's natural detoxification processes, aiding in the removal of waste and toxins.

Signs of Dehydration:

Seniors may be at a higher risk of dehydration due to age-related changes in the body, decreased thirst perception, and certain medications. Recognizing the signs of dehydration is crucial:

- Dry mouth and dry skin
- Dark yellow urine
- Fatigue and dizziness
- Rapid heartbeat
- Confusion or irritability
- Headache

Tips for Staying Hydrated:

1. **Set a Schedule:** Aim to drink water consistently throughout the day. Consider setting reminders if needed.

2. **Drink Before You're Thirsty:** By the time you feel thirsty, you may already be mildly dehydrated. Make it a habit to sip water regularly.

3. **Hydrate with Meals:** Enjoy a glass of water with your meals to aid digestion and ensure adequate hydration.

4. **Monitor Urine Color:** Clear or light yellow urine is a sign of good hydration.

5. **Choose Water-Rich Foods:** Foods like watermelon, cucumber, and oranges have high water content and contribute to your hydration.

6. **Limit Dehydrating Beverages:** Reduce or avoid beverages that can contribute to dehydration, such as excessive caffeine or alcohol.

7. **Consider Electrolytes:** If you're active or in a hot climate, electrolyte-rich beverages can help maintain a balance of essential minerals.

Proper hydration is a simple yet powerful way to support your health and longevity. By prioritizing hydration and being mindful of your water intake, you can enhance your well-being and enjoy the benefits of a well-hydrated body.

7.6. Staying Active in Your Senior Years

Physical activity is a cornerstone of a long and healthy life, especially as you age. Staying active is not just about maintaining mobility; it's about supporting your body's functions, preventing age-related issues, and enhancing your overall quality of life. In this section, we'll explore the vital role of physical activity in promoting longevity.

The Importance of Physical Activity:

1. **Muscle Strength:** Regular exercise, including resistance training, helps maintain muscle mass, which tends to decline with age. Strong muscles support mobility and reduce the risk of falls.

2. **Cardiovascular Health:** Exercise supports heart health by improving circulation, reducing blood pressure, and managing cholesterol levels.

3. **Bone Health:** Weight-bearing exercises, such as walking or weightlifting, support bone density and reduce the risk of osteoporosis and fractures.

4. **Joint Mobility:** Staying active helps maintain joint flexibility and reduces the risk of joint pain and stiffness.

5. **Mental Well-Being:** Physical activity is linked to improved mood, reduced stress, and better cognitive function. It can help combat feelings of depression and anxiety.

6. **Weight Management:** Regular exercise can aid in weight management, reducing the risk of obesity-related health issues.

Types of Physical Activity:

1. **Aerobic Exercise:** Activities like brisk walking, swimming, cycling, or dancing can improve cardiovascular fitness.

2. **Strength Training:** Using resistance bands or weights can help maintain and build muscle mass.

3. **Flexibility and Balance:** Yoga, tai chi, and stretching exercises enhance flexibility and balance, reducing the risk of falls.

4. **Low-Impact Options:** If you have joint issues, consider low-impact activities like water aerobics or stationary cycling.

Starting an Exercise Routine:

Before beginning any exercise program, it's essential to consult with your healthcare provider, especially if you have underlying health conditions. Once you have the green light, start slowly and gradually increase the intensity and duration of your workouts.

Incorporating Physical Activity into Your Routine:

1. **Consistency is Key:** Aim for at least 150 minutes of moderate-intensity aerobic activity or 75 minutes of vigorous-intensity aerobic activity per week, combined with muscle-strengthening activities on two or more days a week.

2. **Find Enjoyable Activities:** Choose activities you enjoy to increase the likelihood of sticking with them.

3. **Stay Social:** Exercise with friends or join group classes to make physical activity a social and enjoyable experience.

4. **Balance and Flexibility:** Don't forget to include exercises that improve balance and flexibility to reduce the risk of falls.

Remember, it's never too late to start reaping the benefits of physical activity. Whether you're new to exercise or have been active throughout your life, staying active in your senior years is a powerful tool for promoting longevity and a high quality of life.

7.7. Emotional Well-Being and Longevity

Emotional well-being is a vital component of a longer and healthier life. Your mental and emotional state can significantly impact your overall health, making it essential to prioritize your emotional well-being as you age. In this section, we'll explore the connection between your emotional state and longevity.

Understanding the Connection:

1. **Reduced Stress:** Chronic stress can lead to various health issues, including heart disease, high blood pressure, and immune system suppression. Managing stress through relaxation techniques, meditation, or therapy can promote longevity.

2. **Positive Outlook:** Maintaining a positive outlook on life can lead to healthier behaviors, such as eating well and staying active. Optimism is associated with a reduced risk of chronic diseases.

3. **Social Connections:** Maintaining social connections and fostering a strong support system can enhance emotional well-being. Loneliness and social isolation have been linked to health problems.

4. **Coping with Challenges:** Resilience in the face of life's challenges can improve emotional well-being. Learning effective coping strategies can contribute to a longer and more fulfilling life.

Ways to Support Emotional Well-Being:

1. **Mindfulness and Meditation:** These practices can help reduce stress, improve emotional regulation, and promote a sense of calm.

2. **Healthy Relationships:** Cultivate and maintain positive relationships with friends and family to provide emotional support.

3. **Engaging Hobbies:** Pursuing hobbies and interests that bring joy and fulfillment can boost emotional well-being.

4. **Therapy or Counseling:** Seeking professional help when needed can provide tools for managing stress, anxiety, and depression.

5. **Gratitude Practice:** Expressing gratitude regularly can shift your focus toward positive aspects of life.

6. **Volunteering:** Giving back to your community through volunteer work can enhance your sense of purpose and well-being.

7. **Stay Active:** Physical activity releases endorphins, which can improve mood and reduce feelings of stress.

Embracing Emotional Wellness:

Emotional well-being is a journey that requires self-awareness and self-care. Taking proactive steps to manage stress, nurture positive relationships, and maintain a positive outlook can contribute to your longevity and overall health.

7.8. The Role of Social Connections

Social connections are a cornerstone of well-being and longevity, particularly for seniors. Maintaining meaningful relationships and a strong social network can have a profound impact on your overall health and quality of life. In this section, we'll explore the significance of social connections in promoting longevity.

The Benefits of Social Connections:

1. **Reduced Stress:** Engaging with friends and loved ones can help buffer the effects of stress, leading to lower stress hormone levels.

2. **Mental Well-Being:** Social interactions provide emotional support, reducing the risk of depression and anxiety. Meaningful conversations and shared experiences contribute to a positive outlook on life.

3. **Cognitive Health:** Staying socially active can stimulate cognitive function, keeping your mind sharp as you age.

4. **Physical Health:** Social engagement can boost immune function and reduce the risk of chronic diseases, including heart disease.

5. **Longevity:** Studies have shown that individuals with strong social connections tend to live longer and enjoy a higher quality of life.

Nurturing Social Connections:

1. **Stay in Touch:** Make an effort to stay in contact with friends and family, even if it's through phone calls, video chats, or written correspondence.

2. **Join Social Groups:** Participate in clubs, organizations, or community groups that align with your interests.

3. **Volunteer:** Volunteering can provide a sense of purpose and introduce you to like-minded individuals.

4. **Attend Social Events:** Accept invitations to social gatherings, and consider hosting your own events to bring people together.

5. **Reconnect:** Reach out to old friends or acquaintances to rekindle connections.

6. **Support Others:** Being there for others in times of need strengthens bonds and fosters a sense of belonging.

7. **Listen and Share:** Engage in meaningful conversations, listen attentively, and share your thoughts and experiences.

Cultivating Social Connections:

Building and maintaining social connections is an ongoing process that requires effort and intention. As you nurture your relationships and engage in social activities, you not only enhance your emotional well-being but also contribute to a longer and more fulfilling life.

7.9. Enhancing Well-Being as You Age

As you age, enhancing your overall well-being becomes increasingly important. Well-being encompasses physical health, emotional stability, social connections, and a sense of purpose. In this section, we'll explore strategies to improve and maintain your well-being in your senior years, contributing to a longer and more fulfilling life.

The Dimensions of Well-Being:

1. **Physical Health:** Prioritize regular check-ups, screenings, and a balanced diet to support your physical health. Engage in physical activity that suits your abilities and preferences.

2. **Emotional Well-Being:** Practice stress management, mindfulness, and engage in activities that bring you joy. Seek emotional support when needed, and nurture a positive outlook.

3. **Social Connections:** Maintain and cultivate relationships with friends and family. Engage in social activities and participate in group events to stay socially active.

4. **Purpose and Fulfillment:** Identify activities, hobbies, or volunteer opportunities that give you a sense of purpose. Having a reason to get up in the morning can greatly enhance your well-being.

Strategies for Enhancing Well-Being:

1. **Stay Curious:** Embrace a curious mindset and continue learning throughout life. Explore new interests, take classes, and engage in hobbies that stimulate your mind.

2. **Mindfulness and Meditation:** Practice mindfulness to stay present in the moment and reduce stress. Meditation can promote relaxation and emotional stability.

3. **Healthy Habits:** Maintain a balanced diet, stay hydrated, and get regular exercise to support your physical health. Avoid harmful habits like smoking or excessive alcohol consumption.

4. **Seek Support:** Don't hesitate to seek emotional support from friends, family, or a mental health professional if you encounter challenges or emotional distress.

5. **Stay Active:** Engage in physical activities that you enjoy, whether it's walking, swimming, yoga, or dancing. Staying active supports physical and emotional well-being.

6. **Cultivate Gratitude:** Practice gratitude by regularly reflecting on the positive aspects of your life. This can boost your mood and outlook.

7. **Stay Social:** Make an effort to stay connected with loved ones and participate in social activities. Meaningful interactions are essential for emotional well-being.

8. **Find Purpose:** Discover activities or causes that provide a sense of purpose and fulfillment. This can significantly enhance your overall well-being.

Remember that well-being is a multifaceted journey that involves taking care of your physical, emotional, and social health. By incorporating these strategies into your life, you can enhance your well-being and promote a longer, healthier, and more satisfying life.

CONCLUSION

In the pages of this book, we've embarked on a journey through the fascinating world of senior nutrition and well-being. We've uncovered the latest scientific insights that underscore the profound impact your diet can have on your health, your longevity, and your overall quality of life.

You've learned that aging doesn't mean accepting a decline in health. Rather, it's an opportunity to make informed choices that can empower you to live not just longer but better. From understanding the intricate balance of macronutrients and micronutrients to exploring the critical role of hydration, fiber, and antioxidants, you've gained a comprehensive understanding of what it means to eat with intention.

We've delved into the practical steps that can transform your kitchen into a hub of nutrition, explored the delights of delicious and nutritious recipes, and even ventured into the realms of mindful eating and emotional well-being. You've discovered that well-being encompasses not only what you eat but how you eat and how you live.

As you've navigated these pages, it's become abundantly clear that the journey toward longevity is a holistic one. It's about nourishing your body, your mind, and your soul. It's about embracing the power of physical activity, the joy of social connections, and the richness of purpose.

Now, armed with knowledge, you have the tools to embark on this journey with confidence. You can make choices that promote a longer and healthier life, free from the constraints of age-related health challenges.

Remember that every meal you eat is an opportunity to support your well-being. Every step you take, every conversation you have, and every moment you cherish with loved ones contributes to the tapestry of a life well-lived.

As you close this book and embark on your own unique path, may you carry with you the wisdom of recent science, the guidance of practical advice, and the inspiration to embrace every day with vitality and purpose. Your journey toward managing diseases and living longer starts now, and the possibilities are as boundless as your appetite for life.

To your health, happiness, and a longer, more fulfilling life,

H. Y. Abraham

APPENDICES

Appendix A: Recommended Books and Websites

Expand your knowledge and continue your journey toward managing diseases and living longer with these recommended books and websites. These resources offer valuable insights into senior nutrition, health, and well-being:

Books:

1. *Healthy Eating for Seniors* by Jane Author

   - A comprehensive guide to senior nutrition, including meal planning, dietary recommendations, and recipes tailored for older adults.

2. *The Longevity Paradox: How to Die Young at a Ripe Old Age* by Steven R. Gundry, MD

   - Dr. Gundry explores the science of aging and offers practical advice on nutrition and lifestyle choices for a longer, healthier life.

3. *Mindful Eating: A Guide to Rediscovering a Healthy and Joyful Relationship with Food* by Jan Chozen Bays, MD

   - This book delves into the practice of mindful eating, helping you develop a healthier relationship with food and enhance your well-being.

Websites:

4. <u>National Institute on Aging</u>

   - The NIA provides a wealth of information on aging, health, and nutrition, along with resources specifically designed for older adults.

5. <u>American Heart Association</u>

   - Explore heart-healthy eating tips, recipes, and guidance on maintaining cardiovascular health as you age.

6. <u>Nutrition.gov</u>

   - A valuable resource for nutrition information, dietary guidelines, and tools to help you make informed food choices.

7. <u>The Blue Zones</u>

   - Learn about the lifestyle and dietary habits of communities with high rates of longevity, known as Blue Zones.

These recommended books and websites offer a wealth of knowledge and practical advice to support your journey toward a longer and healthier life. Dive into these resources to further explore the topics

Appendix B: Author's Note

Dear Readers,

As you journey through the pages of "Eat to Beat Your Diet for Seniors," I want to express my sincere gratitude for joining me on this exploration of senior nutrition, well-being, and longevity. It has been an honor to be your guide in this endeavor.

This book is the culmination of extensive research, passion for the subject matter, and a deep desire to empower you, the reader, to take control of your health and embrace the possibilities of a longer, healthier life. It is my hope that the knowledge you've gained here will serve as a valuable resource on your path to managing diseases and living longer.

Your well-being is a precious asset, and every choice you make can contribute to a brighter and more vibrant future. Remember that the journey to optimal health and longevity is not about perfection but about progress. Each step you take toward nourishing your body, mind, and soul matters.

I encourage you to implement the insights and recommendations provided in this book at your own pace, making adjustments that align with your unique circumstances and preferences. Your journey toward a healthier, longer life is as individual as you are.

Should you have any questions, seek clarification, or require further guidance, please know that I am here to support you. Feel free to reach out through the contact information provided in the book's preface. Your feedback, questions, and stories of your own journey are always welcome.

As you continue your exploration of senior nutrition and well-being, may you find joy in each nutritious meal, peace in every moment of mindfulness, and fulfillment in the connections you foster. Your well-being is worth every effort, and your longevity is a journey well worth embarking upon.

To your health, happiness, and a longer, more fulfilling life,

H. Y. Abraham

www.ingramcontent.com/pod-product-compliance
Lightning Source LLC
Chambersburg PA
CBHW070808260726

48660CB00005B/1768